THE GIRLS IN WHITE

THE GIRLS IN WHITE

Reminiscenses of an Educational Director of the Independence Sanitarium and Hospital School of Nursing

by Vida E. Butterworth

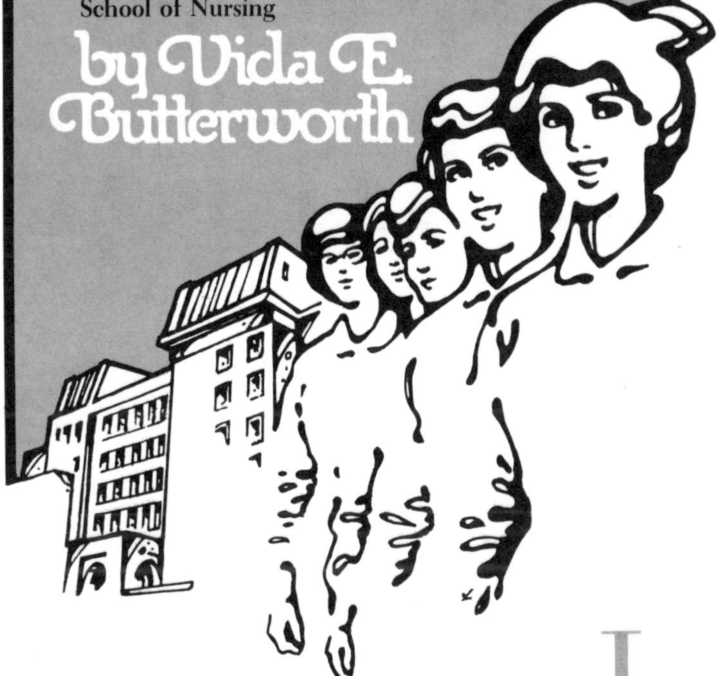

HERALD PUBLISHING HOUSE
Drawer HH
Independence, Missouri 64055

Library of Congress Cataloging in Publication Data

Butterworth, Vida E., 1905-
The girls in white.

1. Independence Sanitarium and Hospital. School of Nursing—History. 2. Butterworth, Vida E., 1905- 3. Nurses—Missouri—Independence—Biography. 4. Independence, Mo.—Biography. I. Title.
RT80.M82I522 610.73'0922 [B] 78-10862
ISBN 0-8309-0230-9

Printed in the United States of America

This book is lovingly dedicated
to all those who were student nurses
at the "San" between 1910 and 1971

CONTENTS

THE GIRL IN WHITE

Stand tall. You must brave toil, study, heartache. Never look back with longing to days of ease, for the firm voice of duty calls: a thousand bed baths, two thousand scrubbings, ten thousand pages of lecture notes. The battle won was never to the weak. Stand tall!

Walk swiftly. Down the halls of pain speed your way. Life and death crown the doorway. Your needles, your vials, your manipulation of tubes will admit one, deny another. Walk swiftly!

Speak gently. Hazy minds and blood-torn bodies grope toward strength. Frighten them not away. Ease their torment with soft words, for who can know in what darkness hides the soul? Woo back from the void with kind tones. Softly . . . softly . . . let His still sweet voice speak through your own with healing power. Speak gently!

Think clearly. Doctors and patients alike depend on you. Marshal your thoughts; look for the hidden symptoms, the elusive signs of danger. For you who daily walk past the ebb and flow of life, there can be no flighty thought, no casual dreams, no absentmindedness. The life placed in your care is worthy of your best. Think clearly!

Live joyously. All the wonder, all the deep, heartwarming love of life is yours. You give your youth, your awareness, your energy to those within these walls. In return, the world is yours. Take its loveliness, its throbbing seasons, its wayside pools, its falling stars. Take the world and all its people. Live joyously!

Enoi Foo Jaynes (1949)

FOREWORD

This book is a history, an autobiography, and a collection of biographies. It tells of various phases of the Independence Sanitarium and Hospital School of Nursing and how these changed through the years that the school was in existence. These changes are not listed in chronological order but in connection with a particular student who went through various aspects of the school at the time of the changes mentioned.

The students described are not exclusive to the phases with which they are connected. Other students and other aspects of the School of Nursing could have been selected. Some have come to mind because of life distinctives.

Indirectly this book of reminiscences tells my story by what it tells about my supervisors, my sister students, my own students. It also reveals the human side of patients, nurses, teachers, supervisors, and doctors. And it tells of the growth of the Independence Sanitarium and Hospital School of Nursing. It deals little with physicians for in "my day" nurses were not permitted to question a doctor or his orders. Times have changed, and now a medical team works for the welfare of the patient, each member of it cooperating with the other, using his or her particular skills to minister to the "whole" patient.

For student nurses who have had similar experiences to laugh over, worry over, cry over, grieve over, be joyful over, and sing over, this book is particularly written. It may be entertaining; it may bring back old memories to those who were educated at the "San" School of Nursing. It may be interesting to the families of former student nurses at that institution.

The fifty years I spent at the San as a student, a private duty nurse, a general duty nurse, an instructor, educational director, patient, and now in my retirement years as a volunteer for the hospital auxiliary have been enjoyable. In fact the San has been my life.

My hope is that readers will enjoy this book, understand the tremendous growth of the San and its various schools, and sympathize with its many problems.

Vida E. Butterworth, R.N., A.A., B.S., M.A.

I ENTER TRAINING AT THE "SAN"

That first morning, May 31, 1926, there were six of us who had lain awake most of the night wondering what tomorrow would be like. We had to don long blue uniforms (six inches from the floor) with white stiffly-starched collars, cuffs, and aprons. We were inspected by the older students to see that we were properly attired. On third floor at the San we stood in line according to seniority until we came to our assigned table at the lowest end of the dining room. The youngest student in seniority had to pour water for all six of us at the table. How her hands trembled. I was asked to say the blessing over breakfast. I was so frightened that I couldn't think. I mumbled, half under my breath, "Our Father in heaven . . . Amen!" I'm sure that the other new students at my table didn't notice and the rest were too far away to hear.

Breakfast was followed by a fifteen-minute chapel period in the dining room. There we sang songs such as "Never Be Discouraged" or "The Lord Knows Why," and listened to a five-minute sermon by an RLDS minister. After the closing prayer we marched out of the dining room according to seniority and as many as could rode the elevator. The rest ran down the stairs to the floor to which they were assigned. We "probies" went to the hospital waiting room on first floor to await our supervisor, Miss Elizabeth Jane Paxton, R.N., a heavyset, black-eyed, black-haired woman. There was never a twinkle in her eyes or a smile on her lips. (Later I learned that she had a "heart of gold.")

She handed a loose-leaf notebook to each of us, then told us to get our fountain pens and start copying the *House Order Book.* By copying this we each would have one of our own. Possessing this was very essential to being a good nurse. Much of it might as well have been in Greek or Chinese. Such words as *hypodermoclysis* and *proctoclysis* left us wondering if we could ever master such a vocabulary.

After supper we were told that we might go back to the Nurses' Home until morning. We went, but we took the *House Order Book* with us, along with paper and pens. By bedtime (10:00 p.m.) we had all succeeded in finishing our copying of the book. The next morning we would be assigned to different hospital wards and begin to do some "real nursing."

My senior student head nurse took me into the supply room to get some newspapers, rags, and soap solution. Then we went to the men's ward where she showed me how to scrub a bed. None of the patients said a word. Nor did I. I couldn't have, with six pairs of masculine eyes staring at me! I wondered how those girls felt who were not used to brothers. When the bed was clean and dry Nurse Hanson showed me how to make a good, tight bed. I was thrilled. At last I had done some "nursing." A new patient might occupy that bed at any moment. I knew he would be comfortable because the sheets were wrinkle-free.

Late in the afternoon an elderly man, a retired RLDS missionary entered the hospital and came back to "my" bed. He brought with him two suitcases, a book-bag, a box, a bundle, and a portable typewriter, which he did not want out of his sight. We tucked them under the bed and felt sorry for the cleaning lady, who would have to move each object before sweeping.

The first bath I gave was to a missionary who had had surgery. I was uncertain, but he said he'd had a bath in bed before and thought that between us we could accomplish our assignment. We did! Several of my first patients were missionaries. They were always cooperative and thanked me for whatever I did for them.

The work was interesting. Meeting the needs of patients on both floors was challenging and rewarding. We "night girls" ate breakfast after work and went to the Nurses' Home for four or five hours of sleep before we had to walk a mile to attend class from 1:00 to 4:00 p.m. Supper was at 5:00 p.m. After that we had an hour and a half that we could spend any way we wanted to as long as we broke no rules or regulations. We were on night duty for a month at a time, seven days a week. Night duty was exciting, especially if babies were born or there were any accidents or emergency operations. At the end of the month we had three days off duty except for class. We were free to do as we wished—again as long as we broke no rules (which were pretty strict). This did not bother me, however, because I had always been expected to be obedient at home.

My family had had a great influence on me. My elder brothers and sisters were, or had been, schoolteachers. They thought I should be one, too, so I became a rural schoolteacher near Dow City, Iowa—but I really wanted to be a nurse. After teaching for two years I decided to enter nursing, and so my family encouraged me.

Fortunately I had saved enough money while teaching to pay my way through three years of nursing education, but just to be on the safe side I entered training in the summertime. If I found that I didn't like nursing I could get back to schoolteaching in the fall.

At one time I planned to enter Jennie Edmundson Hospital in Council Bluffs, Iowa. Then my friend, Argie, transferred to the San at Independence, Missouri, and I decided to go there, too.

I came to the San on May 31, 1926. Argie arrived in August of that year. Another friend, Vida S., came in September. Even so, we were all considered to be in the same class.

Vida J., another friend from near Dow City, Iowa, had entered the San in 1923 and was graduated in the fall of 1926. We were known then as "the three Vidas from Dow City." We even roomed together part of the time.

After the probationary period, we received seven dollars a month pay. Mine always went for shoes and black cotton duty hose. We covered a lot of miles in a month, working fifty-two hours a week.

HEAD NURSES AND SUPERVISORS

By the fall of 1926 no one could have persuaded me to quit nursing for teaching. I was happy. I loved living in the dormitory with the other girls. At home there were only my father, mother, and a brother three and a half years older than I. Much of the time my father was away from home serving in the mission field.

I had always wanted a sister near my own age. In the dorm there were twenty to thirty; we were like a family. I spent more time studying than most of the girls because to me this was serious business. Where I really learned nursing, of course, was in the hospital wards.

When I entered "training" there were only five R.N.'s employed at the hospital.

Miss Gertrude E. Copeland, a graduate of Hahnemann Hospital, Philadelphia, was both superintendent of the hospital and superintendent of nurses. She was a kindly person, interested in the welfare of the patients and the student nurses, but her strict "outer shell" made everyone stand tall and do what she said.

Miss Elizabeth Jane Paxton, a 1918 graduate of the San, was assistant superintendent of nurses and in charge of the pharmacy. She also relieved as operating room and delivery room supervisor whenever the regulars were off duty.

Miss Leta Ralston, a graduate of the 1925 class at the San, was operating room supervisor for a short time until she became Mrs. Goebel and left.

Miss Catherine Stephens, a San graduate, took her place. Miss Stephens also taught operating room technique both in formal classes and during the students' actual operating room experience. She was appreciated as a supervisor, teacher, and friendly adviser.

Miss Ina Cockerton, a graduate of the first San class (1912) was the night supervisor. She was loved by all the student nurses because of her friendly interest and her ability to get the best out of them. On Miss Cockerton's nights off she was relieved by a senior student nurse, usually the one who had highest seniority.

Until 1929 student nurses served as head nurses on each ward. At that time R.N.s were hired as head nurses on the medical floor (first), surgical floor (second), and obstetrical floor (third).

There are three types of head nurses even among students, and I had experience with all three types. These are, first, those who sincerely want to help both patients and students; they are very conscientious and always do their share of the work. Second, there are those who know everything and are convinced that no one else could possibly reach their level of competence. They believe in students coming up the hard way and kowtowing to their supervisors every time they pass in the corridor. Third, there are those who assume that every nurse is as competent as they are and so take responsibility only when the other proves she needs help. Such a person lets a student assume responsibility as soon as possible. The following represented these three types:

Ramona G. (1923-1926)

I remember the day this head nurse (a senior student) was disgusted with us "probies" because we took so long to give a bath, change the bed with the patient in it, clean up a unit, and make the patient comfortable. Ramona G. undertook to give us a demonstration of how to do this whole procedure in *twenty minutes.* It took her *thirty!* We secretly laughed with glee, but outwardly we remained very sober and attentive. We respected Ramona because she *was* a competent nurse, but we were delighted to have her reveal her limitations. We knew, of course, that anyone could be slowed down by various types of patients and by the necessity of meeting special needs.

"Babe" (1925-1928)

I was a probationer and "Babe" was a very domineering student head nurse. (She had won first prize for being the most *ethical* nurse in the School of Nursing.) "Babe" felt it her duty to make every younger student grovel. She actually made extra work for the "probies" because she felt that was what they needed to make good nurses of them.

I was assigned to gather lunch trays, but she gave me so many other assignments to do *immediately* that I failed to get most of the trays back to the diet kitchen in time. As punishment I had to spend my off-duty hours washing and drying trays, dishes, glasses, and silverware and get them back to the kitchen in time to be set up for supper. I *knew* who was boss on our ward. Eventually I even learned to respect her.

Ina C. (1910-1912)

Ina C. was the first graduate of the San School of Nursing. She entered in January, 1910, just a short time after the hospital was opened and she graduated in 1912. As night supervisor she was most efficient, kindly, and helpful. Every night she visited each patient in the hospital. Besides this she was present for the delivery of all babies born between 7:00 p.m. and 7:00 a.m., and any operations or emergencies occurring between those hours.

We all enjoyed being on night duty with her as our supervisor and learned a great deal about nursing because of her guidance.

At the end of our month on night duty she always gave us a party or picnic. The one I best remember was in September, 1926.

On the morning of our picnic breakfast we climbed over a hundred steps from the road near the Missouri River to the limestone cliffs above Cement City about six miles north of Independence. There we built an open fire, boiled coffee (putting an egg in to clear it of coffee grounds), fried bacon and eggs, drank orange juice with bananas sliced into it, and ate homemade cinnamon rolls. We didn't get the least bit sleepy in spite of our hours of duty the night before.

After eating we sat about the fire and Ina told us how her "training" days differed from ours. We could hardly believe that so much improvement could have occurred in only fourteen years. She also told us of her experiences as night supervisor at the old General Hospital in Kansas City where she had worked earlier. There interns and residents did all operations that had to be done at night. One night a man came in with an injured leg that required amputation. After the patient was under the anesthetic the young doctors lacked the nerve to sever the leg so Ina completed the surgery successfully herself.

When I was no longer a probationer, Miss Paxton called me into the drug room late in August and gave me three unlaundered caps and six bibs. She said as soon as they came back from the laundry I could wear them. I was so proud!

This was not like the elaborate capping ceremony of student nurses in later years. The first to be officially capped in public was the class of 1938. The students' mothers were invited to the capping ceremony in the afternoon and then stayed on for supper in the dining room.

In still later years capping exercises were held in various churches. Eventually there were banding ceremonies also in which student nurses received service stripes at the end of each year.

I have many memories of my early years at the San. Among them is the time a senior student relieved the night supervisor and found that the kitchen help had left very little food for the night nurses. Out in the hen house, which belonged to the hospital, were quite a number of chickens. When Willard, the night watchman, was elsewhere, two students crept out and grabbed three chickens and cut off their heads with a hatchet. The hatchet (only evidence of the bloody deed) was wrapped in a towel and hidden under a pile of laundry in the second floor linen closet by another student. The chickens were then picked and cleaned and fried. Willard, who had heard suspicious noises in the region of the hen house, inspected the area very thoroughly but could find no evidence of foul play, so he went back to bed. That night the nurses had all the chicken they could eat, and they never forgot the adventure of acquiring it.

Another night, when Ina was on duty and the kitchen help left no food for the night nurses to warm up, she cooked a duck she found in the icebox. The next day she and all the rest of the night nurses were in trouble because we had eaten the duck that had been a gift to a patient and was to have been cooked for her the next day. Ina took all the blame for that and replaced the fowl.

When I was on third floor night duty I had to give the mothers milk at bedtime to insure their having enough milk to feed their babies. I fed them chocolate milkshakes made with cream skimmed off the top of the big urn. Ice cream was allowed to melt into it before mixing. Those mothers really enjoyed their bedtime snacks.

One night when Ina was off duty, the girls asked me to make fudge. (Fudge is my specialty—I have been making it since I was seven years old.) After I had my third floor patients put to bed, I went to the kitchen and started making the candy. In walked the day supervisor, Elizabeth Jane Paxton. I expected a long lecture, but she merely said, "If you want to stay out of trouble you had better bring me a sample of that as soon as you are off duty." I acquired new respect for Elizabeth Jane that night; it was nice to know that she was human, too.

There was another time when I bought materials for fudge making uptown so I could treat the girls at the dormitory. Nelle decided to help me. We had boiled it and were beating it when a pair of cockroach legs surfaced. Nelle thought I was fooling when I said, "We can't eat this because it has a roach in it." She grabbed the pan and stirred up the body. Without a word she went out the back door and poured the candy under the bushes behind the nurses' home. I had no money to buy more materials to make another batch and all of the stores were closed anyway, so we sneaked back to the hospital and "borrowed" the necessary ingredients. That candy was found to be exceedingly good to all who tasted it.

Years later when I was teaching at the San and the student nurses did not get to go home during the holidays we would have a candy party the week before Christmas. Each girl was permitted to make candy for herself, her boyfriend, or her family at home. The girls enjoyed this very much. The custom was discontinued after the students began having two-week Christmas vacations. (Increased costs and increasing numbers of students also influenced this decision.)

Good things happened, and I call up happy memories of those days when Ina was our supervisor. She was well liked by everyone and respected as a competent nurse and supervisor.

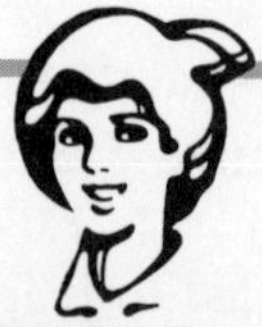

WHEN I WAS HEAD NURSE

I well remember my first month as a student head nurse. It was in January 1927. I had had no prior experience or classwork in obstetrical nursing, so being head nurse on that floor was especially difficult for me. At that time Miss Copeland and Miss Myrtle Grapes, our instructor, made rounds through the hospital (every floor) once a week to see how well each department was kept up, what kind of nursing care was being given the patients, how well the individual student nurses were doing, and especially how well the student head nurse was functioning. I remember that all the nurses on the floor, the day before the inspection, had spent every spare moment cleaning, polishing, and shining the equipment so that it would be spotless for the inspection. It was just our luck that there were several deliveries the night before inspection and a couple early in the morning so that all our cleaning and polishing had been in vain. When the two inspectors came at 9:00 a.m. (our floor was the first to be inspected since this morning they started at the top and worked their way down) the equipment was a mess. We hadn't been able to clean up after the deliveries because they came too close together.

In the report in which the inspectors gave the results of their surveys I was severely reprimanded for mismanaging the floor. This was hard to take because I had done everything humanly possible to have my floor in order, but to no avail. I was determined to quit training where I was not appreciated and go back to Iowa! The only trouble was that I had just had my eyes tested and had ordered new glasses. When I paid for them, I did not have train fare home, so I had to stay and make the best of it.

I remember on another occasion when I was a student working the night shift on first floor, I was the only nurse for the twenty-four patients in the ward. I also had to answer the switchboard in the office and admit new patients. This particular night we had a delirious patient in the women's ward and I had orders to watch her closely. I did this between answering patients' lights, taking temperatures, giving medications, and tending the switchboard.

Once when I had to answer the switchboard and was gone several minutes this patient disappeared. The window by her bed was wide open. I called the night supervisor who said, "Find her!" I went outside around the building, but couldn't find her. In the meantime the night supervisor called the police. In just a few minutes they brought back our patient clothed only in a hospital "shorty" and a T-strap.

Another night when I was acting as night supervisor over the whole hospital, we had five children brought in from a burning home. They were fourteen-year-old twin girls, a five-year-old boy, a twelve-year-old girl, and a nine-year-old girl. We had to put on wet tannic acid dressings, which took hours. The little boy was so badly burned that his thigh had popped open just like an overdone roast. He died before morning. One twin, the twelve-year-old girl, and the nine-year-old girl died before I came back on duty the next night. Such a tragedy! The one twin who did get well was subject to epileptic seizures. (Why do parents go away from home leaving children alone?)

Another time while I was serving as student head nurse on first floor (medical) we had a Mexican suffering from pneumonia in the men's ward. (This was before the days of antibiotics.) He was a heavy drinker, and in spite of the "spirits of frumenti" (whiskey) which we gave as medication, he developed delirium tremens. He needed to be in bed, but we could not keep him there. Even when he was in a straitjacket and secured tightly to the bed, he would get out. So we quit putting him in a straitjacket, locked both ward doors, and left him alone in the ward with five empty beds.

One time I went back, unlocked the door, and carefully looked around to see where he was. There he was—sitting on the floor playing with the twenty-four wheels he had carefully removed from all of the beds in the ward. Finally he recovered both from his pneumonia and the "dt's." He had a rugged constitution when he was struck down by the microscopic pneumococci.

Another patient I cared for that I will always remember was a man who, while cranking his car, was pinned between it and another car. His abdomen was crushed and his whole gastrointestinal tract reacted violently to this trauma. The only relief for him came with a narcotic hypo, swallowing a half-inch stomach tube to wash his stomach, and getting a "gas" enema. At first we had to do this every two hours. He is the only patient I ever knew who begged to have his stomach washed. Eventually he got so he'd do both the stomach wash and the enema on himself without help. All the nurses had to do was bring him the equipment. He, too, recovered.

Still another patient I remember well when I was student head nurse on third floor was a woman seven months pregnant. She had threatened to deliver early so the doctor had sent her to the hospital. I was working at the chart station when the light over Ward 300 came on. I hurried back to Mrs. D, who asked to be put on the bedpan. (Remember, I had had no previous obstetric classwork or experience.) She gave a big grunt, ending in a sharp cry, and I hastened to look under the cover. There in the bedpan was a small baby in a bag of fluid with a membrane over its face. I reached down and pinched a hole in the membrane and out came a small but perfect baby boy. In the nursery he tipped the scale at three pounds and twelve ounces. He was so sturdy he was able to go home with his mother. "The powers" were not too happy about having a baby born without benefit of doctor or R.N.; I was just thankful that my ignorance had not harmed either mother or baby. Of course, again I was "hauled on the carpet" for letting the baby come without getting the patient to the delivery room or having the doctor present; the woman, however, was so happy over having such a sturdy little boy that she didn't care how she got it.

Another time when I was in charge of the obstetric floor at night I had a young student on duty with me. I went off duty to sleep in an empty room and warned the student to be sure and wake me if any new patients came in.

About midnight I was wakened by the student saying, "Hurry! We have a new patient and I'm afraid she will deliver any minute." I arrived at the delivery room door just in time to see one of the baby's legs protruding. When I saw this I knew that soon the cord would be pinched off, so if we didn't get the baby's mouth and nose out in six minutes the baby would die for lack of oxygen. I had seen this kind of delivery before. I poured alcohol over my hands, took hold of the baby's leg, put the other hand inside the mother and my fingers in the baby's mouth. Gently twisting the whole baby I luckily pulled it out of the birth canal. When it began to cry I knew the baby was okay.

I received quite a "dressing down" from the doctor when he came. He said, "Didn't you know that baby was breech [came lower body first] and could have died if it hadn't gotten oxygen right away?" Of course I knew—that was why I acted so spontaneously when I saw the situation. The doctor said, "You should have called me when the patient came in." I knew that was what had been done, but I also knew better than to "talk back" to a doctor, so I just bit my lip and said, "Yes, sir. I'm sorry, sir," and walked away.

It was during these early years that I learned something quite important that I never would have suspected—that is, babies can be tricky. I could sit at the chart desk and when a baby began to cry I would get up and go to the nursery door. There would not be a "peep" out of a single baby. When I went back to my charting and closed the nursery door, the baby would start crying again.

To fool the baby I would go into the nursery again, where all was silence. I would walk to the door, close it, and remain in the room. Almost instantly the crying would begin again. This time I would see who it was—change his diaper, pick him up, put him over my shoulder, pat the bubbles from his tummy, or give him a drink of water. Then all would be quiet again.

There were more patients that were made memorable to me as a student head nurse. Each experience was unique. There were other duties besides caring for patients, however. I had to keep an accurate inventory of all instruments and hospital equipment, night and morning. If anything came up missing I had to look until I found it—or pay for it. I had to assign the care of patients to the other student nurses assigned to my ward, and assign other nurses to clean—dressing trays, procedure equipment, bedpans, urinals, water sterilizers, dishes used by "infectious" patients, linen closets, bathrooms, and workroom. I also had to order patient drugs, floor stock drugs, dressings, and other such supplies; supervise the care of all patients on the ward; see that all necessary charting was done on each patient; see that cotton swabs, cotton balls, and dressings were prepared for sterilization; wait on the physicians as they called on their patients and help with treatments; see that the medicine chart was accurate and up-to-date; and try to enforce visiting hours. The life of a head nurse was a busy and fulfilling one.

MEMORABLE PERSONALITIES

FAYE FRANKLIN

Faye had been an Iowa schoolteacher, but in 1918 she decided to change her vocation and become a nurse. Because of her membership in the RLDS Church she chose to come to the "San."

Faye was graduated from the School of Nursing in 1921. When I first knew her she was employed to give care in the home to patients who carried Metropolitan Life Insurance or to patients who went home from the San still requiring some nursing care to hasten their complete recovery.

As a student I spent one month traveling with her—bathing the mother while she bathed the baby, changing a dressing, removing stitches from an incision, and other nursing procedures. Most of us students felt it a real privilege to get this "taste" of public health nursing under our beloved Faye's supervision. We mostly made the house calls in the morning; after lunch she taught us in the hospital wherever there was an empty room. If none were vacant, we would put some of the dining room tables together and sit around them. In those days nurses were very versatile.

We also learned massage in the dining room. For this we removed the tablecloth, spread a bath blanket over the table, and used another for a cover. We became quite expert as masseuses. We should have, because when we arrived at the dorm after twelve to fourteen hours of nursing we often recuperated by giving each other massages.

After some time elapsed Faye moved to Columbia, Missouri, where she worked at the University Hospital for twelve years and at Ellis Fischell State Cancer Hospital for six years.

She returned to Independence as medical supervisor on third floor in 1946 and worked there four years. From 1950 until 1966 she took charge of central supply. Even then she had not had enough of nursing and continued to work part time at Resthaven from 1965 until just recently.

San nurses organized their Alumnae Association about 1915 with Ina Cockerton as the first president. This was formed to provide a means of keeping track of San graduates and their employment. It also was dedicated to providing some financial support to the School of Nursing and to the hospital.

The alumnae met every month or two except during the summer. Besides doing business and having a social hour they sponsored many moneymaking projects to purchase things needed at the San. Here are some I can remember:

1. Purchasing the first movie projector for the school.
2. Furnishing the Alumnae Lounge in 1943 when the

first three floors of the hospital were completed and occupied.

3. Providing a new movie projector and three nursing films for the school.

4. Giving $3,000 to the hospital for expansion in the 1950s.

5. Helping finance the celebration of the thirty-fifth, fiftieth, and sixtieth anniversaries of the San and the School of Nursing.

6. Raising money for a hospital chapel. This was the major project of the Alumnae from 1950 to 1976. It started out with a Hawaiian luau on the Campus which netted about $5,000. Members sold many things to raise funds—nuts, steak knives, vegetable cutters, candles, stationery, cards, vanilla, and baked goods.

The chief moneymaking projects were bazaars, chili and soup lunches and suppers, bake sales, and white elephant sales.

In 1961-62 Bishop G. Leslie DeLapp pushed to get a gift from the church toward the building of the chapel. The 1964 Conference appropriated $25,000 for that purpose and in 1966 another $10,000.

All during these years Faye Franklin served as chairman of the Chapel Finance Committee. Mrs. Blanche Craton was chairman of the Chapel Committee. Her husband, Darrell, was of invaluable help in selling tickets, purchasing supplies at wholesale cost, and doing a lot of manual labor. Since he was so well liked he was able to sell many tickets and even to get many needed supplies donated or bought at cost.

There is now an Interfaith Chapel in the new hospital towers finished in 1976. It provides a setting in which patient, nurse, doctor, chaplain, and visitor may come to pray, meditate, or worship.

Services are held in the Chapel every Sunday morning at 10:00 a.m. It is colorful and beautiful. Just being in it makes one want to worship God.

On the curved wall, printed in gold letters, are these words:

We Believe. . .

In God as the source of love and life and truth

In Jesus Christ as the Personal Revelation of God

In the Holy Spirit as God's presence with and in us

In the Human Soul as body and spirit

In the Ultimate Health of Salvation as perfect wholeness through divine grace.

It is a joy to see the chapel and learn the significance of each piece of artwork—the doors, the pews, the color scheme, the organ, the pulpit, the Communion table, the outside tile figures.

Since Faye Franklin chaired the moneymaking committee, the Alumnae chose to have her portrait painted and hung on one of the outer walls to represent all nurses who helped raise funds for the Chapel.

Another project of the Alumnae was to send out birthday brochures to all graduates of the School of Nursing and invite them to donate to the Chapel Fund a penny for each year that the Independence San had existed. Of course, most of them sent more. This raised considerable revenue through the years.

Still another Alumnae project was its *Newsletter*, which carried information about the alums, where they were, and what they were doing. At first it was published and sent out every six months; then it became an annual periodical, twenty-four to twenty-six pages long, and required an assembly line to get it ready for mailing.

I started this project in the 1940's and served as editor. The last copy was published early in 1977 after the Alumnae Association was disbanded.

The Alumnae Association also held annual dinners at which some person important to the group was honored. This received considerable publicity in the newspapers. Honorees have been:

1952—Gertrude E. Copeland and C. H. Allen, M.D.
1961—Fred W. Hink, M.D.
1962—Charles F. Grabske, M.D.
1963—Stanley L. Green, M.D., and
John R. Green, M.D.
1964—Charles E. Nickson, M.D.
1965—Faye Franklin, R.N. (1921)
1966—Raymond F. Gard, M.D.
1967—Myrtle Grapes Quitmyer, R.N. (1924)
1968—Mabel M. Faulkner, R.N. (1932)
1969—Everett L. Saunders, M.D.
1970—Vance E. Link, M.D.
1971—Nelle Morgan, R.N. (1930), and
Vida Butterworth, R.N. (1929)
1972—Chaplain Donald Harvey
1973—Margaret McKevit, R.N. (1955)
1974—President W. Wallace Smith
1975—Bishop G. Leslie DeLapp

The honorees' close relatives were invited as guests. In addition to the dinner there was a program including a presentation of the biography of the person or persons being honored.

On October 30 and 31, 1976, the Alumnae Association held a homecoming at the Sanitarium. Members were welcomed by Earl Horton, executive director of the hospital, who told them how proud he had always been of the San grads even before he came to Independence. He had had some of them on the staff of the hospital in California where he was director. He said he had always found them to be dependable, to have good initiative and judgment, and to be empathetic with the patients and with those with whom they worked. He always had been glad to hire a San graduate.

Miss Margaret McKevit, R.N., B.S., M.S., now director of the School of Nursing at Louisiana University, was the principal speaker.

At a business meeting it was voted to disband the Alumnae Association as soon as it could be done legally, and to turn over any money left after settling all bills to the Myrtle Quitmyer Scholarship Fund of the RLDS Professional Nurses Association for nursing scholarships.

In the evening a banquet was held in the Hospital Auditorium with President Blanche Craton and Vice-President Betty Taylor as emcees. The classes sat together at tables so they might reminisce more easily.

As former educational director of the School of Nursing I recognized the San graduates who had been members of the ISH School of Nursing Faculty. Cited for her service to the Alumnae Association was Blanche Craton (1929) who had served as president of the Alumnae Association longer than any other San graduate and who also had served as chairman of the Alumnae's Chapel Committee since its beginning. As a classmate of Mrs. Craton's I was asked to present her with an engraved silver tray.

On Sunday morning, October 31, a service of recognition and dedication was held in the new Interfaith Chapel. Leslie DeLapp spoke on "Chapel Goal—A Dream." "This I Remember" testimonials were given by Faye Franklin, R.N. (1921), Mabel McKevit, R.N. (1931), Nora Kyger, R.N. (1948), and Evangelist Robert Farnham.

President Maurice L. Draper spoke on "Chapel—A Reality" and gave the prayer of thanksgiving and dedication.

Music was provided by Mary Jo Kittinger, R.N., and Phyllis Fortman, R.N., with Jeweldean Spillman at the chapel organ.

The Chapel cost over $135,000, of which the Alumnae raised over $100,000. The rest was appropriated by the church.

The Alumnae Association board held a final meeting on May 25, 1977, and the association was disbanded in the summer of 1977.

In the October 17, 1975, *Independence Examiner's* "Outstanding Clubwoman Contest," Faye was named "Clubwoman Emeritus."

MYRTLE GRAPES QUITMYER

Myrtle Grapes of Strawberry Point, Iowa, was born in another century. Before entering the San she was a bookkeeper, stenographer, general office girl, and photographer. A graduate of the school of nursing, class of 1924, she was older than most of the students who came to the San so it was quite natural that she should become an instructor.

Prior to 1926 the student nurses were taught in their hours off duty by Faye (1921) and Eva (1924) Franklin and staff physicians. Dr. W. E. Messenger, Dr. C. E. Krimminger, Dr. Stanley L. Green, Dr. John R. Green, Dr. W. W. Hobbs, Dr. Charles Keown, Dr. Calvin Atkins, Dr. Stuart Gillmore, and Dr. C. H. Allen were among those who served as instructors then and in later years.

By the summer of 1926 it became important to have a full-time faculty member to insure that all students would receive adequate education so that after completing the course they would be eligible to take the Missouri State Board of Nursing Examinations and become registered nurses. To become qualified to take charge of the educational program of the school, Myrtle Grapes attended Northwestern University. I can remember when Miss Grapes came to the San in September 1926, after returning from summer school at Northwestern. She organized the classes in bacteriology, psychology, hospital housekeeping, history of nursing, ethics, chemistry, mathematics of drugs and solutions, nursing procedures, and *The House Order Book.* She also attended the doctors' lectures, tried to guide them so that all aspects of their subjects would be covered, and gave the student examinations in those subjects. Miss Grapes was a very efficient and busy instructor.

I remember one time she called me aside and said, "You have the hands of a lady. You'll never make a nurse!" I didn't let that bother me because I knew those hands had done a lot of hard work in our truck garden, berry patch, and orchard as well as keeping house and doing the family baking for eight to ten people. I was just lucky to have the type of hands that did not show the hard work they had done. (Now after fifty-one years my hands are gnarled with arthritis and cupped in because of shortened tendons so I can no longer give back rubs.)

Miss Grapes taught at the San from 1926 to 1930, then became an instructor at Christ Hospital in Topeka, Kansas, for one year. In September, 1931, she married Irvy Quitmyer, widower of a longtime friend. For a while she did private duty nursing at the San, but after her husband died she rejoined the staff as instructor in Fundamentals of Nursing and Mathematics of Drugs and Solutions.

Mrs. Quitmyer had a tremendous influence for good on all the students. They respected her forthrightness, her knowledge, and her skill. Students practiced their nursing procedures over and over again to perfect them so Mrs. Quitmyer would give her stamp of approval.

When the Recreation Building was completed in 1953, Mrs. Quitmyer wrote a pageant depicting the history of nursing since its beginning. This was presented for the benefit of the community by the student nurses and hospital employees; all who participated dressed in vivid costumes of the time represented.

Mrs. Quitmyer had many talents and characteristics that added to her usefulness in the School of Nursing. She was persistent in anything she undertook. I remember when my class graduated (1929) she wrote the words to our class song. She also helped us plan and carry out "Senior Sneak Day." We all took off work and went out to have a good time. Of course, it was sanctioned by the school.

When "Mrs. Q" felt that teaching Fundamentals of Nursing was too hard for her she resigned from that position and took over as librarian for the School of Nursing. She continued to teach the Mathematics of Drugs and Solutions because she seemed to have the ability to "get math across" to the students better than most other instructors. For one thing, she never gave up. She never conceded that a student "just couldn't learn math."

She retired as librarian and later moved to Resthaven where she was very happy. Several other retired San nurses were there, and she organized them into a class. They had some lively discussions that made their lives more interesting. "Mrs. Q" could be depended on to stimulate and enliven any environment.

When she became very ill, she was transferred to the San. She died in the institution where she had served so efficiently as an instructor during her active years.

Many of us still miss "Mrs. Q" and wonder what project she is engaged in while she awaits the Millennium. We feel sure that wherever she is she is working in a worthy cause.

"Mrs. Q" was always properly uniformed and groomed and demanded the same of her students. She was interested in the students' uniforms, the design of which changed through the years. The following excerpt is taken from the "School of Nursing History—1909-1959" which she wrote:

From 1910 to 1912 the student nurse wore a cotton dress with a "kitchen" apron of any design or color that pleased her personal taste during her first three months in the "training school." At the end of three months she donned a cap with very little ceremony, a blue and

white striped uniform with a high collar and long sleeves, and a white apron with bib. It was considered most professionally proper that those long sleeves be rolled down neatly before entering the dining room. Elsie Barnett Wombles in 1915 secured the privilege of allowing the students to wear short sleeved uniforms with a cuff on the sleeve.

The first cap was made of organdy with a gathered frill in the back. From 1920 to 1933 the uniform was blue chambray with stiff white collar and cuffs and a full gathered white apron with a bib. Later, a cap with a straight fold in front was worn. The present cap was adopted in 1926. This has a pointed cuff when it is folded back. It may be the same cap style, but it, too, has undergone changes in the way the cuff is folded back. The one-piece white uniform was adopted in 1933; black shoes and hose continued to be worn with the uniform until 1943, when the change was made to white shoes and hose. The blue and red cape became a part of the uniform for the graduating class of 1929. There were those who thought the cape should be purple and gold (church colors); but the nurses wanted the blue and red cape with the red lining, so blue and red were selected after the nurses petitioned the Board of Trustees that it be so.

The black band on the cap for the graduate nurse was proposed by the Alumnae and adopted by the school in 1926. In 1956 something new was added to the uniform to distinguish between the grades of student nurses. When a student is seen in a plain white cap, everyone knows that she is a freshman in her first year in the school. The student nurse with one royal blue stripe on the left-hand corner of the cuff of her cap is a junior in the second year. The two stripes of royal blue on the left-hand corner of the cuff of the cap indicate the senior student nurse. Nursing instructors give the senior student her two stripes, and the seniors, in turn, give the junior students their stripes. The Banding Service is a significant step in the progress of the student nurse's education.

One of the *Sanilogs*, dedicated to "Mrs. Q.," contained these lines:

> We, the students of the Independence Sanitarium and Hospital School of Nursing, wish to dedicate this *Sanilog* to Mrs. Myrtle Quitmyer, who has been a guiding light and an enthusiastic teacher not only to us but also to those many who preceded us. Her life has been and is truly a life of human service. Her sympathetic understanding and kind heart have endeared her to us and many others.
>
> So for these reasons and others too numerous to mention we affectionately and humbly dedicate this *Sanilog* to you, Mrs. Q.

GERTRUDE E. COPELAND

Gertrude E. Copeland was a graduate of Hahnemann Hospital School of Nursing in Philadelphia, Pennsylvania. She served as an Army Nurse in both the United States and France during World War I. After a period at hospitals in Pennsylvania following the war, she became superintendent of the Independence Sanitarium and Hospital on January 3, 1923. She was also superintendent of the School of Nursing.

At that time the San had only sixty beds and the school only twenty-four student nurses. Under her superintendency the hospital grew to over 200 beds (plus 34 nursery cribs) when all of the floors of the "new" hospital were completed in 1943. The School of Nursing grew to 114 students in 1969.

When she retired in 1953 she had served the hospital exactly thirty years. During her superintendency the hospital and school made tremendous strides as well as increasing in the number of patients and students. New departments were formed, new classrooms were opened, and the quality of the school was improved. She served during the critical times of the depression and World War II. Under her direction the San School of Nursing received national accreditation and, during the war, participated in the United States Cadet Nurse Corps training program.

She was honored on January 3, 1948, upon completion of twenty-five years of service, at a reception given by the Hospital Board of Directors, the School of Nursing, the Medical Staff, and the Nurse's Alumnae Association. The board resolved

that we extend our sincere admiration, respect, and gratitude for what she has accomplished for our institution, for service indeed valuable beyond estimation, and our sincere wishes that she may live long to enjoy a release from the stern responsibility to which for so many years she has been faithful and true.

That a copy of these resolutions be suitably engrossed for delivery to her, to be signed by each member of the board and

That as a further mark of our appreciation and regard, we give to Miss Copeland a watch of quality in keeping with her loyalty to the best traditions of her profession and the office she has so ably magnified since January 3, 1923.

During Miss Copeland's regime the old 1909 three-story building was remodeled as a Nurses Home. The hospital grew as the community grew, and so did the School of Nursing.

Miss Copeland's chief hobby was the making of wedding veils and bridal coronets for friends, former students, and hospital employees. She spent half of her life at the hospital and her friends were many. Another hobby was dressing dolls with complete wardrobes, plus a wedding gown and veil.

She cared for her mother, Mary E. Copeland, until her death. Her mother was an excellent cook and cooked most of the meals served when they had dinner guests. Gertrude always said she couldn't cook, but after Mother Copeland's death she still invited her many friends to luncheons and dinners. She was a marvelous hostess, being able to sense which people would be congenial dinner guests.

Miss Copeland almost always had the top of her desk covered with neat piles of papers, magazines, and books. She was practically never at a loss to find anything. She would select the right pile and carefully pick each item up, turn it over, lay it down, smooth it, and go on to the next until she found the thing she wanted. All the time she was looking she would be talking to those in the room. She was usually very kind, but she could be quite sharp if the person to whom she was speaking was not meeting with her approval.

When she sat talking to another woman she would rub her left knee. And when she wanted to emphasize a point she would tap the other person's knee in a friendly way. When I was a student I was frightened in her presence. She was always so dignified, but she had a rather keen sense of humor. On her half-days off duty she enjoyed going to Kansas City to shop.

After I became instructor at the school and after Mother Copeland had died, Gertrude and I went on a number of vacations together—Philadelphia to visit her sister-in-law; Ithaca, New York, to visit my brother and sister-in-law; Kentucky, to visit her niece; Atlantic City and Miami Beach to attend hospital or nursing conventions. She was good company.

Gertrude Copeland knew how to spend money wisely, both personally and for the Sanitarium. She kept the San doors open during the depression! In 1932 she employed the entire graduating class of twelve because there were no jobs available elsewhere for them.

Miss Copeland stated many times that she never felt ashamed of the education given the girls at the San. She told of many instances when she had heard how competently some graduate from the San had performed in her hospital or community or church. She was proud of "her nurses" and always was delighted to hear what they were doing for the good of the world.

She belonged to the Greater Kansas City Hospital

Council, serving two terms as its president and four terms as secretary.

Upon retirement she was presented a console television set as a token of appreciation by the staff doctors.

ELVINA RICHMOND

Elvina Richmond came from the island of Tahiti with Apostle and Mrs. Clyde Ellis in 1923 to enter nurses' training at the San. Tavita Petis, another Tahitian girl, came with her. Both were graduated in 1926.

After graduation Elvina chose to do private duty nursing, which meant that she cared for one patient twenty hours a day. She was supposed to sleep on a cot in her patient's room at night in order to be available when necessary. She also was supposed to have from 1:00 p.m. to 5:00 p.m. off duty each day. During that time student and head nurses would assume the care of this patient. For twenty hours of nursing care per day private duty nurses received the sum of six dollars. If the patient was very ill the private duty nurse seldom took time off even in the afternoon, remaining with her patient because she wanted to do so.

At one time Elvina and another nurse were hired to care for a very ill patient. One night when Elvina was on duty the room became very chilly so Elvina turned the radiator on full heat and sat near it with a blanket wrapped about her shoulders. The next morning she had a burn on her foot where it had touched the radiator. That didn't mean much to the rest of us. After all, a burn was just a burn. But to Elvina this was no simple accident. As an Islander she knew of anesthetic leprosy, a disease fairly common there. In this disease the nerve is so involved that it does not pick up pain sensations. Elvina was panic-stricken. She *knew* she had leprosy.

Even in her terror she was a lady. After all, royal blood flowed in her veins. She waited for the doctor to make his rounds that morning to show him her foot and to tell him of her fears. Dr. K______, the pathologist, consulted his colleagues and the diagnosis came back just as Elvina had feared: anesthetic leprosy.

She was immediately admitted to Room 106, the best in the San. Her diagnosis was kept secret except to a very few for fear the townspeople would not permit the San to "harbor" a leper. She was placed in very strict isolation. No one could enter the room without mask, gloves, and isolation gown. A special nurse was assigned to care for her with one other to relieve her on her days off. My friend, Argie, was assigned, and I was the relief nurse. We enjoyed caring for Elvina. She was cheerful and tried hard to mask the pain she suffered when we gave her treatment "shots" (chaulmoogra oil) deep in the muscle. This medication burns like fire when given and causes abscesses afterward. Elvina appreciated what we did for her. Argie and I read everything we could find about leprosy. We discovered that the disease was not highly contagious, especially in our temperate climate. We also learned that the incubation period for leprosy was twenty-five to thirty years and that it practically never was contracted by a doctor or nurse caring for a leper. We had a little doubt in the back of our minds, however. One trouble was that we could not know for sure if we had contracted the disease from Elvina until between 1951 and 1956. To us that seemed eons away.

Arrangements were finally made to transport Elvina to Carville, Louisiana, the only leper colony in the United States. A U.S. Public Health Nurse accompanied her to Carville in a special railroad compartment. (When I was teaching at the San I always devoted a little time to the study of leprosy even though it was uncommon in our part of the country. For years I took *The Star*, a little newspaper published by the patients at Carville to disseminate new information about the disease and its care. I always told my students about Elvina.)

Eventually Elvina was transported from the United States to a leprosy island in the Philippines. There she assumed the role of a nurse at the leprosarium. She kept in touch with some of us by correspondence that was sterilized before mailing. Some time after I was graduated I had a letter returned marked "deceased." Later I learned that Elvina did not die of leprosy but of tuberculosis. (The mycobacterium which causes leprosy is very similar to the tuberculosis mycobacterium.)

Elvina kept up the best traditions of the San: "Help others as much as you can and as long as you can." She was a credit to the school and to the nursing profession.

Eventually Elvina's memory slipped to the background of my mind because of more pressing matters, but I continued to take the newspaper from the lepers at Carville. There has been a big change in the treatment of leprosy since those days. A series of drugs known as the sulfones are being used to treat lepers. Practically no state requires lepers to live out of their own homes, because the disease was discovered not to be that contagious, and lepers can recover. When Elvina was treated at the San all the furniture in her hospital room was burned so that there would be no fear hanging over anyone who was a patient or an employee at the San. In fact, that was the room in which I was a patient when I had a submaxillary abscess and erysipelas. My temperature reached 106° and I heard a report over the telephone that I was not expected to live through the day. Word was sent to my mother, who lived in Iowa; this was almost never done when a student was ill. Brothers Floyd McDowell and F. Henry Edwards administered to me; to this I credit my recovery. I felt that I was spared because God had special work for me to do.

Even in solemn moments there can be humor. After seeing only doctors or nurses in isolation gowns I found it comical to see ministers wearing them. They didn't quite have the "hang of it." I say this with no disrespect, for I have long held these two men in high regard and feel honored to have worked with them in religious, hospital, and School of Nursing projects.

In 1961 Elvina again came to mind when we received an application to enter the San School of Nursing from Elvina's niece, Theresa Richmond from Papeete, Tahiti. Theresa knew little about her aunt, because Elvina had died before Theresa was born.

It was nice to have another Tahitian in the school. In addition to being a good student Theresa was talented. She demonstrated some of her native dances and songs at variety shows and school programs put on by the student nurses. The San School of Nursing that Theresa Richmond discovered was vastly different from the one her aunt had known. It had grown and changed and improved. Theresa had some difficulty with her lessons because she spoke French and Tahitian much more fluently than English, but the students and faculty were glad to help her. She was graduated in 1964, took the state board exams in Missouri, then returned to Tahiti. There she practiced nursing in her native land—a thing her aunt was never permitted to do.

In 1976 an RLDS missionary who was transferring from Tahiti to France stopped in Independence. When I asked him about Theresa he said that she was the nurse in a large tourist hotel, that she was well and doing good work.

GLADYS HEIDE

When I entered training at the San I met about twenty-five other student nurses—probies, juniors, and seniors. Among those was Gladys Heide, a tall, raw-boned, good looking, enthusiastic junior with a very positive view of life.

As students came off duty at 7:00 p.m. they were in a hurry to get ready for their dates. In the whole Nurses Home, however, there were only two bathtubs for use by the twenty-five students, and each girl had to bathe before leaving the dormitory in order to get rid of the anesthetic and antiseptic odors. Hence there was always a rush for the tubs. Heide never even tried to get a tub; she simply found a sink that was not in use, stripped, and took a sponge bath. We saw her sponging her weary body so often that we named this type of ablution the

"Heide bath." Needless to say many other students than Heide made use of this type of quick cleanup.

Once when I was on night duty I had Heide's boyfriend as a patient. He had had a tonsillectomy that day and was to be in the hospital overnight. About 2:00 a.m. he rang and wanted to go to the bathroom, so I took him there in a wheelchair. We were no sooner in the bathroom than he raised up and vomited what seemed like quarts of dark clots and bright red blood. Then he fainted, stretched out full length on the bathroom floor. I couldn't get him up and back to bed alone so I called the night supervisor to help. Who was relieving Miss Cockerton that night? Heide! In no time at all we had the patient in surgery with Dr. Stanley Green tying off the bleeders. I was really frightened but Heide knew exactly what to do and she did it without any sentimental involvement. This was the mark of an excellent nurse.

Heide is no longer living but when I think of her I wonder how many cheerful and efficient nurses God has need of to carry out his plans where there is supposed to be no more illness.

I like to think that all of the nurses there are serving others in any way they can. I would say that those who have developed compassion, tenderness, accuracy, interest in the welfare of others, empathy, social and psychological skills should continue to be helpful in the Hereafter.

FLORENCE HANSEN GRABSKE

After completing high school Florence worked at the National Cloak and Suit Company. She entered the San School of Nursing in September, 1925. This was the same year that her sister, Katie Hansen Frederickson, was graduated from the San.

Florence, a blue-eyed blonde, was well liked by everyone—by her classmates because she was a good speaker and had a keen sense of humor, by the younger students because she was always helpful and never tried to play jokes on them, by her instructors because she was intelligent, by her supervisors because she followed instructions carefully, by her patients because she gave them good nursing care, and by the physicians because they could trust her judgment.

She was graduated July 29, 1928, which indicates that she must have worked overtime to complete her training in less than the full three years. After graduation she served as a private duty nurse, caring for patients in the hospital and in their homes. During this time she relieved the operating room supervisor for her vacations. Early in the thirties she became full-time operating room supervisor at the San.

She was very efficient in this role, thinking of the patient's welfare and providing the necessary instruments, linens, and equipment that the surgeon needed during the operations. She taught students well both in operating room technique and in private demonstrations of how to scrub, set up for, and assist the surgeon in all types of operations. She also taught them self-sufficiency so that they could assist the surgeons at night without her.

In 1940 Florence married Dr. Paul Grabske, a dentist. She did not work long at the hospital after her marriage. Instead she assisted her husband in his dental office. She remained a very active member of the School of Nursing Committee, however, and served as secretary for the committee until the school was closed in 1971.

JENNIE GUNLOCK CADY

Jennie, one of my classmates, was a brown-haired, gray-eyed lass—little but mighty. Jennie always seemed to minister to the sickest patients, those without friends or relatives, those with incurable diseases, the mentally disturbed. She had compassion for the most forlorn, the disfigured, the homeless, the downtrodden. She was well liked by her patients because she was a good, conscientious, dependable nurse. Because of these attributes she also attracted many boyfriends.

There were few evenings that Jennie did not have a date. She was generous in sharing her boyfriends with those of us who did not have any. We shared many a ride to the movies and late snacks with Jennie and her dates.

Occasionally when a group of us yearned for excitement we would get some of the boys to climb from the porch up a tree to attend one of our card parties. We kept blankets over the windows and doors so that "Mother Thomas" could not see the light. (Lights were to be out at 10:00 p.m., and playing cards with male company in our rooms, especially after hours, was definitely against the rules—all of which made the games much more fun.) These were perfectly respectable parties. We often had snacks sent from home which were shared with everyone present. After the card game was over the boys would depart the same way they came.

Since I had no boyfriend, I most often invited my nephews who were just slightly older than I.

Jennie was married early, shortly after graduation. She did little nursing until her two daughters were grown, then she worked in a doctor's office. Jennie and her husband, Kenneth, have been very involved in church work since their marriage. They now live on a small acreage near Springfield, Missouri, near their two married daughters, six grandchildren, and one great-grandchild.

Jennie has lived up to her promise in training of being a persevering, cheerful, helpful, courageous helpmate. She is another San graduate who has been successful as a nurse, neighbor, wife, and mother. I regret that I have not had more opportunity to be with her during the fifty-one years since we entered the School of Nursing back in 1929.

Many San students have been exceptionally popular with persons of the opposite sex, and gradually there has been an easing of regulations concerning dating. In later years boys who wanted to date nurses were known as "lounge hounds." They would come to the Nurses' Lounge and stay until they found a girl willing to go out with them.

Many of the girls who had steady boyfriends spent their dates in the School of Nursing Library where each studied his or her own lessons. These were usually couples who intended to marry as soon as one or the other completed school. The one who was graduated first would help put the other one through. Since nursing was a three-year course, the girl usually finished first and would work to finance her husband's education. It was known as "PhT" (Putting Hubby Through).

By 1944 students were permitted to marry during the last six months of training (with the consent of parents, School of Nursing Committee, and faculty). By setting such a date it was thought that if a girl became pregnant she would still be able to complete her nursing course at the regular time. A rule was made that a student nurse could not be on duty after she was more than five months pregnant. The San was the first School of Nursing in the Kansas City area to allow student nurses to marry and still continue training.

Eventually students were permitted to marry at any time during their nursing course if they had the written consent of their parents, were interviewed by the Hospital Chaplain, and obtained approval of the School of Nursing Committee and the faculty. By the late sixties many graduating classes had from one third to one half married students. If a girl became pregnant she was out of the school beginning with the sixth month of pregnancy until her six weeks postpartal examination (or whenever her obstetrician gave her permission to return).

The school admitted its first married student, Doris Beckstrom, in 1949. (Her biographical sketch appears later.)

As well as "letting up" on the marriage requirement, the committee also gave consideration to older women.

Formerly the age requirement for student enrollment had been between seventeen and thirty-five years of age. This rule was later amended to read "older by special permission of the School of Nursing and of the Missouri State Board of Nursing." The first of these older women to enter the School of Nursing was Catherine Bath Davis. She had begun training in 1926 with my class but left to marry. In 1949, when most of her children were on their own and she was a widow, she reentered, completing her course in 1952 as Catherine Bowers. Often the younger students called her "Grandma." Being older, but not an authority figure, she gave words of advice that often were more acceptable to a student than if they came from administration or faculty. Since she did so well in nursing, a number of other older women were allowed to enroll. This was a far cry from the qualification of a student in 1910, 1926, 1939, or 1945. Many improvements were made between 1926 and 1952.

BLANCHE MINTON CRATON

I don't remember Blanche too well in training because although we were classmates we did not live on the same floor at the Nurses Home. I do know that she was a good student with a keen sense of humor and a steady boyfriend who was both handsome and good-natured. At that time he was working as a milkman to pay his way through pharmacy school.

She was a competent student nurse who was sincerely

interested in the welfare of her patients. I liked to be assigned to a ward with her because she always did her share of the work.

I remember that Blanche made a high average on state board exams. She was not only intelligent but shrewd. In those days, the exams contained essay type questions. Out of the twelve we were given we had to answer ten. One of the things we were asked to do was describe in detail the anatomy of the entire leg—bones, muscles, blood vessels, and nerves. For some reason Blanche couldn't remember the anatomy of the leg, but she could remember the arm. So she said to herself, "I'll just go ahead and describe the arm instead of the leg. They'll think I just misread the question and give me a good grade." She was correct. She made 98 on the test.

Blanche and Darrell were generous and often provided transportation for other student nurses while they were dating. I'll never forget the night of our graduation rehearsal when we were on our way from Children's Mercy Hospital where we were on duty until after 7:00 p.m. Rehearsal was in Independence at the Stone Church at 7:30 p.m. Miss Copeland warned us that if a single one of us dared to be late we might not get to graduate.

We were speeding so as not to be late when behind us we heard a police siren. We were stopped for speeding and escorted back to the Police Station at Independence Avenue and Benton Boulevard. They asked us if we were going to a fire. What saved us was the brand-new blue and red capes in the back seat of the car. We were released and allowed to go on our way.

Blanche and Darrell were married the June after she

completed training. Several of her classmates participated in the ceremony. One, Irene Engstrom, was in Blanche's wedding one night and the next night was the bride at her own wedding to Paul Shearer.

The Cratons did not have children of their own, but they aided in the growth and development of many nieces, nephews, grandnieces and nephews, and the children of friends.

Blanche has been a member of the Independence Sanitarium Hospital Alumnae Association since her graduation in 1929. She has almost always been an officer, committee chairman, or committee member. For eight years she was president of the Alumnae Association. She was serving in this capacity when the association voted itself out of existence. There was no need to continue after the school closed in 1971 because no "new blood" would be coming into the organization.

NELLE MORGAN

Before coming to the San Nelle was a saleslady in a department store in Albia, Iowa.

She was one of the original six students who entered "training" at the San June 1, 1926, before there was a full-time instructor. Nursing procedures were taught by older student nurses.

Nelle had a severe illness and had to take a leave of absence to recuperate. At that time student nurses at the San were having 550 hours of classwork and 1,096 days in the nursing course. Because of her illness Nelle was a student for 1,655 days, although she spent 559 of them either as a patient in the hospital or at home in Iowa recuperating. At that time students had to make up all time missed due to illness or any other reason. (Later in the school's history they did not have to make up sick time unless it was an excessive number of days.)

Nelle was graduated with the "Centennial Class" of 1930, with commencement exercises being held in the main chamber of the Auditorium. After graduation she worked as a private duty nurse for one year. Then she joined the staff at Menorah Hospital in Kansas City, Missouri, where she worked for three years. After that she became a Kansas City school nurse and served as supervisor for a time. She also spent some time in Utah as a Public Health Nurse.

In 1943 the Hospital Board of Trustees hired Miss Morgan to relieve Miss Copeland (who was not so young any more) of her responsibilities with the School of Nursing and to oversee the bedside care of all patients in the San. This gave Miss Copeland time to take care of the various phases of hospital business—student and school costs, cost of hospital care to the patient, purchasing of hospital and school supplies, etc.

In her role as director of the School of Nursing Miss Morgan faced a number of changing situations. Many students graduating after the forties were married before completing their nursing course and several even had children.

Miss Morgan was the students' best friend, whether they were in trouble at the school, having family problems, making poor grades, or just not getting in at midnight on late leaves. She could talk "straight" to them, give sound advice (which they may or may not have taken), and deal with worried parents.

I remember what students (and faculty members) used to say when they were told, "Miss Morgan wants to see you." Invariably the reply was, "What have I done now?" It was she who upheld the discipline and dignity of the school.

Some of the students who particularly resented discipline would write in from three to five years after graduation and say, "I couldn't see at the time that what you were insisting on was right, but now I am so glad you stuck to high nursing principles."

Miss Morgan and I always laughed together about a rumor that existed about her office. The students were supposed to have said to one another, "Be careful when you go to Miss Morgan's office—she keeps a tape recorder in the bottom drawer of her desk which she turns on when she is interviewing students." The only tape recorder the school owned was far too big to go in any desk drawer; it would have taken a third of the top of her desk.

The students dedicated their 1964 *Sanilog* to her with these words:

In grateful appreciation for your years of service to our hospital and our nursing school and for the constant example you are to us in the nursing profession we dedicate this Sanilog to you "our nurse of the year" and always, Miss Nelle Morgan.

One way she managed to get her work accomplished was through the organization of many groups. These included the following:

1. Faculty
2. School of Nursing Committee with representatives from various areas of the church and the community.

(Having this committee made up of representatives from so many areas facilitated solving many problems of the school.)

3. Hospital supervisors
4. Hospital head nurses
5. Licensed practical nurses
6. Auxiliary personnel (practical nurses, ward secretaries, and nurse aides)

With some of these groups meeting once a week, every two weeks, or each month, there were meetings going on a good bit of the time.

Miss Morgan could and did delegate responsibility. She gave people jobs to do, checked to see they hadn't forgotten, and then expected them to have the report when it was called for. In this way she was able to accomplish a great deal of work.

Miss Morgan visited all patients in the hospital in order to know firsthand how well they were being cared for. Her Director of Nursing Service received 6:45 a.m. and 2:45 p.m. reports of patients and their condition. There were also written reports of the patients for the three daily shifts.

The San had some of the best publicity of all health institutions in the Kansas City area after Miss Morgan became Director of Public Relations in 1968. She was acquainted with all of the available avenues of publicity and knew personally many reporters. She had been at the San long enough to know its history thoroughly and had ideas as to how to present the publicity. If she did not know she sought help.

During these years she was not just working in the hospital and school. She had many other responsibilities:

a member of the Governor's Advisory Council on Hospital Construction from 1946 to 1950; president of the Missouri State Board of Nursing from 1947 to 1956; and president of the Missouri State Nurses' Association from 1944 to 1946. She was listed in the fifth edition of *Who's Who in the Midwest.* In 1962 she was honored by Theta Sigma Phi at its annual Matrix Dinner as a "Woman of Achievement" in the Kansas City area. In 1963 she was named the "Outstanding Nurse in Missouri" by the Missouri League for Nursing and received the All State Gold Medal Award. In 1971 the Nurses' Alumnae Association honored her for her years of work at the San and the School of Nursing.

In 1973 this nurse of forty-seven years retired. All who worked with her were proud of her and proud of the School of Nursing and of the hospital where she so adequately used her talents.

SHIRLEY BUTLER

Shirley came to the San in September 1927 from Inman, Nebraska. She was a good student, dependable, sweet-tempered. She not only had great strength of character but a sense of humor. While a student nurse she took it upon herself to see that one of her classmates completed her nursing course. Almost every night when this student returned to the Nurses Home she would pack her suitcases and plan to leave training. And just as often Shirley would unpack them. The girl remained to finish her nursing education.

One day the work on a particular hospital floor was especially busy; almost all beds were filled. Every doctor arrived at the same time that morning, and it seemed to the girls on duty that there were not as many nurses circulating around as there should be. All of a sudden Shirley realized that she had not seen a particular one for an hour or so and decided to investigate. She went up and down the halls looking in each room. As she approached one she heard a *creak, creak* of the floor boards. When she opened the door and looked in she saw the missing student sitting in a rocking chair, rocking back and forth. Shirley spoke rather sharply: "What are you doing in here? Don't you know we are extremely busy out there on the floor?"

The student replied, "Well, I finished *my* patients and was so tired I thought I'd rest a bit. It seems to me one should be allowed rest when tired." Shirley continued to look at her sternly, so she got up and came out to join the fray. I never heard of this kind of incident happening again.

While Shirley was affiliating at Children's Mercy Hospital in Kansas City, Missouri, she contracted diphtheria and was very ill for some time. In spite of her illness she was only a month late in completing training, finishing September 30, 1930.

After graduation Shirley worked as a private duty nurse in Independence for one year. After that she went to Menorah Hospital in Kansas City, Missouri, to do general staff nursing. She was a Kansas City School Nurse from September 1937 until 1943 when she came to the San to be in charge of the student health program and to teach medical nursing and sociology. Before this she had attended Michigan State University along with Nelle Morgan. Shirley also took some classes at the University of Kansas City to help her in teaching courses at the San.

She had been hired to teach in the School of Nursing because so many doctors had been called into military service that those remaining in Independence were too busy to teach classes. From this time on more and more faculty members were employed as the number of students increased with the coming of the Nurse Cadet Corps. The number of patients being treated in the hospital also increased; this required more nursing personnel. When Miss Morgan's load became too heavy for her to handle alone Shirley was employed as Assistant Director of Nursing Service.

Late in the 1960s Miss Butler became Director of Outpatient Referral Services. As such she served as coordinator between patient, doctor, relatives, and outside agencies that might care for patients in the home, or other agency. She made the final arrangements to get the patients out of the hospital and to the place where they could get the kind of care they needed. In these different positions she had to develop new skills and new categories of knowledge.

Shirley had tragedy in her life. Her father died shortly after the family moved to Independence. Her sister, Mary, died of cancer, leaving two young sons. Later in the same year her sister, Anne, died of cancer, leaving a daughter and son. (Anne, a 1943 graduate of the School of Nursing, was Operating Room Supervisor for a short time.)

Shirley's mother served as a "housemother" at the

Nurses Home for a while before the school closed. About the time of Shirley's retirement her mother became bedfast, so Shirley cared for her until her death.

Shirley is now a member of the Hospital Auxiliary and serves as a volunteer at the Information Desk, gift shop, or ICU.

Through all the vicissitudes of life she has remained optimistic. She has many friends because she *is* a friend.

MARGARET CHAPMAN ESLER

Margaret entered the School of Nursing in September, 1927, after being graduated from William Chrisman High School in Independence. Students liked her because she had a good sense of humor, and patients appreciated her because she was empathic and anxious to meet their needs.

After graduation from the San she went to Chicago for a course in pediatric nursing at Cook County Hospital.

She did some private duty nursing in Independence then went to Hawaii. There she met her husband, who was in military service. Margaret was living in Honolulu at the time the Japanese bombed Pearl Harbor and had some harrowing experiences. One day her husband, who was flying out of Hawaii, took off on a mission and was never heard from again. Although the officials tried and tried to trace him they never succeeded.

Since Margaret was pregnant she decided to return to Independence where her parents lived. Her son, George Esler, was born at the Sanitarium.

Realizing she must rear her son by herself, she obtained a Bachelor's and Master's degree in Public Health Nursing. She served as a school nurse in Kansas City, Missouri, until her retirement. After that she seemed to be busier than ever, belonging to many organizations including the Nurses' Alumnae (as long as it existed), the Doll Club, a quilting group, and art groups. She paints china, pictures, and doll faces. Her home is filled with antique furniture.

Her special hobby is restoring antique dolls and dressing them according to their era. She also likes to visit and help care for the aged, incompetent, and others who have health problems. She is generous with her time, her money, and her talents. Her son is married now, and one of her great joys in life is her grandson.

MABEL FAULKNER

Mabel entered the nursing school in September, 1929, and was graduated November 12, 1932. She had been a teacher in the Kansas Public Schools for eight years so she was older than most San students. She was sincere, kindly, and dependable.

After receiving her R.N. she served as a general staff nurse for four years at a Chicago lying-in hospital. In 1936 she returned to the San as night supervisor, a position she held until 1942. From January to June, 1941, she took over my duties in the classroom while I finished work on my master's degree.

In 1962 Mabel began teaching obstetrics to the students. She also served as obstetric supervisor until 1971.

As such she counseled each mother about caring for herself and the baby after they went home.

She was responsible for starting the prenatal classes for expectant parents and taught them weekly. Often as she travels about town she meets someone who says, "Aren't you Miss Faulkner? You took care of me when I had my baby. I remember how kind you were."

In 1968 she was honored by the Alumnae Association. She also was named "Employee of the Year" at the San in 1969 and went on to win the "Employee of the Year Award" of the hospitals in the greater Kansas City area.

The students dedicated the 1955 *Sanilog* to her. In it they wrote:

> **To you, Miss Faulkner, because of your concern in our education, the endless patience you employ in teaching us, and your interest and helping hand in our activities, we dedicate the 1954-55 *Sanilog* with our affection and respect. We warmly appreciate these qualities which we find so constant in you and the inspiration they give to us serves as one of the stepping stones to our accomplishments.**

In 1969 the *Sanilog* was again dedicated to her, with this tribute:

> **Miss Mabel Faulkner, a Truly Wonderful Person . . .**
>
> **One who nourished us and caused us to grow by implanting knowledge, wisdom, and truth within our beings.**
>
> **Advising justly, assisting readily, defending courageously—accepting us for what we are.**
>
> **By being a mother to many people—loving all infants as her own; instructing the new mother, holding the new babe; you have not loved one child, but all children. By giving your love to others, you have become an inexhaustible treasury.**

Throughout the years Mabel proved her loyalty to the San, the School of Nursing, the church, and the community.

She was honored at a reception when the diploma

school closed. Mayor Phil Weeks presented her a plaque and "key to the city." The employees gave her a money tree.

Following her retirement Mabel did volunteer work at the Northeast Jackson County Mental Health Center in the day activity center program for over two years. She is now a member of the Hospital Auxiliary and works as a volunteer at least one day a week at the Information Desk or in the Volunteer Office.

Mabel has belonged to all of the professional nursing organizations ever since she was graduated (or since they were formed). She served as treasurer of the Alumnae Association until it was disbanded in 1977.

She was involved in planning celebrations for all of the school and hospital anniversaries since she was graduated; therefore these celebrations are listed as a part of her biography.

Thirty-Fifth Anniversary

The San School of Nursing was thirty-five years old January 10, 1945. At this time open house was held in the school, its classrooms, and laboratories.

Student nurses displayed lab exhibits, trays of special diet foods, posters, sample classroom projects, microscopic slides of various kinds of bacteria, anatomy charts, and sample term papers. They also put on nursing demonstrations. After touring the exhibits guests were served refreshments.

Golden Anniversary

In 1960 the San School of Nursing was a half century old. Open house was held in the new Education Building on February 28, 1960. This building was begun in April, 1959, and completed in February, 1960. Financing was made possible by funds secured from the Hospital Construction Act, General Conference appropriations, and San School of Nursing Day contributions.

The ground floor housed the library, science laboratory, lecture room, and offices for the educational director, her secretary, and one instructor. Other classrooms and instructors' offices were on the ground floor of the original building (which later became the Nurses Home), and the assembly room was located on the ground floor of the 1943 hospital building.

Skits were presented by student nurses dressed in uniforms of different periods of the San School of Nursing—1910, 1915, 1926, 1934, and 1940, including the summer and winter U.S. Cadet Nurse Corps uniforms.

Many changes had occurred during the fifty years. In 1910 four students had been enrolled at the School of Nursing. In 1960 there were 119.

The first graduating class (1912) consisted of one graduate, Ina Cockerton. In 1960 there were thirty-nine graduates and a total of 632 alumnae.

In 1910 the nurses' residence was on third floor of the hospital. In 1960 the school had the following residences:

105 West Truman (housing 81 students)
108 North Park (housing 12 students)
1413 West Truman (housing 6 students)

The rest of the students were on affiliation.

In 1910 there were only a few books in the hospital corridor. In 1960 the library—a spacious, well-lighted room seating 40 students—contained 3,000 volumes.

In 1910 there were no classrooms. In 1960 there were four lecture rooms, two ward classrooms, and a science laboratory.

In 1910 there were no organizations to accredit schools of nursing. In 1960 the School of Nursing was fully accredited by the Missouri State Board of Nursing and the National League for Nursing.

In 1910 there were no recreational facilities; in 1960 a building which would seat 200 guests was available. It was equipped with stage, fireplace, sports equipment, kitchen, volleyball court, and outside oven.

In 1910 there were six physicians on the medical staff. In 1960 there were eighty-five staff doctors and dentists.

In 1910 there was no student government; in 1960 an active student association of which each student was a member was functioning. The student council planned and administered student activities and extraprofessional affairs with the cooperation of individual faculty members.

In 1910 the hospital and twenty beds, one operating room, no delivery room or nursery. In 1960 it had 202 adult beds plus 34 nursery cribs, five operating rooms, two delivery rooms and one "lying in" room, a nursery with three divisions, an emergency room, a physical therapy department, a pathological laboratory, X-ray department, and a medical records department.

The Alumnae Association was organized in 1914 with Ina Cockerton as president. By 1960 the alumnae met once a month. Through the years the association contributed to the growth of the school by financial contributions, assistance in recruiting students, and disseminating publicity concerning the hospital and school. In 1960 the president was Margaret Walker Rowe (class of 1948).

The Fiftieth Anniversary Committee consisted of Nelle Morgan (chairman), Vida Butterworth, A. Neal Deaver, Evelyn Directo, Alice Dyer, Stella Earnshaw, Florence Grabske, Bishop H. L. Livingston, Myrtle Quitmyer, and Margaret Walker.

Sixtieth Anniversary

The 1970 celebration consisted of a week of special day observances for the following:

1. Students and faculty
2. Hospital employees
3. Hospital board of trustees, School of Nursing committee
4. Hospital supervisors and head nurses
5. The Alumnae Association
6. The general public—friends of the students, the School of Nursing, and the hospital.

When the school was closed on May 22, 1971, 1,046 nurses in fifty-eight classes had been graduated. (There were no graduates in 1913 and 1935.)

Mabel Faulkner, as a San employee and treasurer of the Alumnae Association, was active in all of these anniversary celebrations.

DOROTHY SCHOLL ARNOLD

Dorothy was a tall, quiet, blue-eyed blonde who came from a farm near Shamrock, Missouri. She was almost always to be found at the edge of the crowd with little to say unless directly questioned. Then she would answer smilingly as though pleased someone thought her important enough to ask.

A conscientious student, she was graduated from the San School of Nursing in 1936 and left Independence. I do not know where she went or what type of nursing she did until after World War II was declared. At the San we received information that Dorothy had enlisted in the Army Nurse Corps in 1940.

The next I heard of Dorothy was when she returned to the United States late in February, 1945. She had served in the Philippines, Bataan, and Corregidor and had been a prisoner of war of the Japanese from December 24, 1941, to February 3, 1945.

While moving their sick and wounded and hospital supplies to Bataan the Americans often had to get out of the trucks and jeeps and hide in the ditches to avoid being bombed by the Japanese. On one trip they arrived at Camp Limay on the beach of Bataan at noon, where there were ten Army barracks and two warehouses. These were used as hospitals, nurses' quarters, kitchen, and supply buildings. Dorothy spent thirty-nine days on the beach and in the woods of Bataan, eighty-five days on Corregidor, and seven weeks at the Santo Catalina Convent in Manila locked in a room with sixty-seven other nurses. While there she was ill with malaria for two weeks. The rest of the time she was in Santo Thomas prison.

The Japanese stripped the American soldiers of everything valuable—knives, guns, jewelry, etc. Dorothy managed to keep her watch. While she was in bed with malaria the Japanese were taking the watches off the nurses while they were in bed. Since Dorothy did not want to lose hers she stuffed it under her pillow. The Japanese would never leave a nurse without a watch when she was "on duty," but often they liked the nurse's watch better than the one they had so they would insist on trading. (Frequently the watch the nurse received would be more valuable than the one she gave up.)

While nurses were on duty they were always under the guard of Japanese soldiers. Whenever a soldier approached a nurse she rose to her feet and bowed from the waist down. In general nurses were well treated, but American officers and soldiers were roughed up.

Nurses were confined to quarters except from six to seven in the evening when they could roam around the enclosure and talk with other nurses. Almost all Americans lost from thirty to fifty pounds while prisoners. This they rapidly regained when they came back to American quarters on February 3, 1945. Dorothy said that food was brought to prisoners in dirty garbage buckets, but they ate it anyhow.

To keep up the morale of the nurses on Bataan they organized clubs for sewing, reading, gardening, sports, etc. They made over their worn-out clothes and even learned to knit things from tattered garments that had been raveled out to provide yarn.

Just before the Americans returned to Bataan someone sent in a lot of fresh fruit—pineapple, mangoes, and bananas. Dorothy said that never in her life had anything tasted as good. Christmas of 1945 was her happiest Christmas. She laughed and cried for joy because she knew the Americans were coming.

On her way home she paused long enough in Kansas City to participate in a Red Cross Rally. She told how they had received Red Cross packages in December, 1943. These contained powdered milk, canned meats, butter, canned fruits, and chocolate.

Dorothy said that the Americans never doubted that McArthur would return.

At home in Independence she had six weeks to rest up before again reporting for duty. She spent the time eating, sleeping, and visiting.

Dorothy was generous in sharing her war experiences. She always spoke in a quiet, unassuming manner. She said she was proud of the training she had received at the San.

After the war she married an army officer, and I did not have the privilege of meeting her again. I will always think of her as one of the pluckiest nurses ever graduated from the San. I am proud of her and of her work.

LUCY MARIE NELSON LAND

Lucy Marie entered training in September 1934. She came from a closely knit farm family near Gower, Missouri. The Nelson children entered various professions. Lucy Marie became a nurse; Bertha Mildred, a dietitian; one of the boys, an M.D.; and another, an "educated" farmer.

Lucy Marie was sentimental. I remember some of the girls telling of her getting a letter from home, and as she read it tears started rolling down her cheeks. One of her classmates said sympathetically, "What's the matter, Lucy? Is your family having difficulties?" Lucy sobbed, "Papa just sold our old mule."

Lucy Marie was a good nurse both academically and clinically. She had great empathy for her patients and their relatives. She made the highest average of any member of her class on state board exams and immediately became assistant head nurse on the Medical Floor—a position she held for three and one-half years. In 1942 she became the second instructor in the School of Nursing.

In the summer of 1943 she went to New York City to study at Columbia University. She returned to the San, married Helmut Land, and taught until 1945 when she resigned to have her first baby. The Lands eventually had three children—Garland, Jennifer, and Daniel.

Lucy Marie did group nursing at Research Hospital in Kansas City for two years. Then the family moved to Lamoni where she served as college nurse while her husband attended Graceland (1951-53). In 1954 Lucy Marie became a Graceland student herself. Then she returned to the San as medical-surgical clinical instructor. She was assistant medical supervisor for six years and did private duty nursing for nine years. Most of the time since then she has done either office nursing or assisted the doctor in orthopedic surgery. She has led a full life that has benefited her family, her church, her community, her students, and a great many sick people.

Lucy Marie was in the first class of San students who had town parents assigned to them. This was a successful facet of the school. Town mothers had been provided for Graceland girls from "far away." This gave the student a place to go away from the college and someone to talk with when she needed advice or a quick cure for homesickness. Great care was taken to try to match up mothers and daughters with similar interests. Later it was felt that student nurses also needed town fathers and perhaps sisters and brothers, so the emphasis was placed on families rather than mothers exclusively.

Junior students were delegated to plan an evening reception for new students and prospective town families. This was a "dress-up" occasion. Most town parent-nurse daughter combinations worked out very well, and many lasting relationships were formed.

MARGERY SHEEHY BOONE

Marge's sense of humor was as big as all outdoors. She came by it naturally. Both her father, John, and elder brother, Almer, were pranksters all their lives.

Marge entered the San School of Nursing in the late summer of 1935. She was a member of the first class I taught all three years. We were serving our probationary period together—she as a student and I as an instructor.

At this time classes were held in the unfinished basement of the "new hospital" (started in 1930 but left uncompleted for years). The building was just a shell connected to the old Sanitarium by an underground tunnel. In this basement we had a nursing laboratory with six to eight hospital beds and equipment, a dressing room, a rest room, a science laboratory and a formal lecture room with a blackboard (literally a board painted black and mounted on two enema standards).

The walls dividing these rooms were made of sheets hung from wire and pinned at strategic points.

Marge enjoyed her jokes in class—as we all did. I had a chance to play a joke on her at Christmastime her first year in the school. The students had their party in the Stone Church Annex. At the end of the program I came in dressed as Santa Claus with a bag of gifts on my back. These gifts were especially prepared for each student. For instance, one girl named Dorothy received a two-quart bucket of salt water—the tears I had collected during her first two weeks in the school when she cried continuously.

Several weeks after the Fourth of July Marge had lit a firecracker in the pathological laboratory where she was working. Inside that small room the sound was greatly magnified. A number of people were frightened and Marge was called on the carpet for her irresponsible behavior. My Christmas present for her that year was a firecracker which I lit, after calling her name, and threw across the room, thus startling her and everyone else present. (Such irresponsibility! When I think about that episode I realize God protects us in our foolishness as well as in our more serious moments. Sparks could so easily have set fire to the cotton around that Christmas tree or to my Santa Claus beard. In fact the whole Stone Church Annex could have gone up in flames.)

Marge was an excellent student and nurse. Her sense of humor was an asset to her, her patients, her fellow workers, and her family. Marge has held many responsible nursing positions besides rearing a family.

Marge married Dan Boone and lives in South Bend, Indiana. (Her son, Dan, Jr., is a veterinarian.) Marge has just become an OR/RR instructor. Previously she was a member of a cardiac surgery team for years in one of the local hospitals.

DORIS ELIASON CASTER

Doris Eliason came to Independence from Montana in the fall of 1939 with her family. Since her mother was quite ill Doris had more problems to contend with than those associated with "training." She managed these very well and was an outstanding student both in classwork and in sensing and meeting her patients' needs. She was rather quiet, but not shy.

Among her "first and lasting" impressions of the San and the School of Nursing are the following:

She remembers her introduction to the Nurses Home at 1215 West Van Horn Road. While she was on the third floor unpacking she was visited by two bare-chested "upper classmen" from second floor. If they planned to shock Doris their mission was accomplished.

When the school was young a student nurse had a day added to her training if she was detected chewing gum on duty.

Many a girl was sent home to lengthen her uniform when she came on duty with it too short. The standards changed, of course—in 1926, six inches from the floor; in the 1940s, ten inches; in the 1950s, fourteen inches; and in the late 1960s and 1970s, to the bend of the knee—or full length pant suits. Nursing styles were affected by fashion, although more slowly than the avant-garde.

In 1940 no radios were allowed in the students' rooms at the Nurses Home. Later when TV became popular, sets were not allowed in student rooms because the wiring in the old San that became the nurses' residence would not carry the extra load. There was, however, one at each nurses' residence. At the old San there was one in the students' lounge (where boyfriends might enjoy it too) and one in the Student's Recreation Room on second floor (where the students might watch it without being fully dressed).

The housemother answered many telephone calls, notifying the students if they were at home or writing out a message if they were out. When a student left the nurses' residence she had to sign in a book when she was leaving, where she expected to go, and when she expected to return. Some students felt this to be an infringement on their rights.

The housemother rang a bell at 10:00 p.m. to dismiss visitors and "tell" the girls to go to bed. All lights were to be out at 10:30, but the students discovered that if they put blankets over the doors and windows they could keep the lights on. Usually they did this so they could study for tests far into the night.

At 6:00 a.m. the bell rang again to indicate that it was time for them to get up, dress, and go to breakfast so they would be ready for compulsory Chapel at 6:45 a.m. before going on duty at 7:00 a.m.

Since living was rather communal, steps often had to be taken to curtail the activities of a certain few to protect the majority. For instance, one girl played the piece, "My Buddy," so much on the piano that someone hid the music under the rug.

The year Doris came initiation was rough. Each probie was soaked with water, had the initial "P" painted on her forehead with silver nitrate (which came off only as the skin peeled), and was fed undercooked beans. Other years probies had to eat donuts soaked in ice tea served from bedpans. (The bedpans were brand-new and had never been used, but the probies didn't know this.) A favorite was to give the probies pills which caused their urine to be orange, red, green, or blue, then ask them to bring urine specimens to the laboratory the next morning. This caused much consternation. Usually when they found out they resolved to try it on the probies next year.

Occasionally probies had to dress like children, and when they met an upper classman they had to bow to their superiors.

After the Recreation Building was built, the probies were taken there by their "big sisters," and each probie had to go to the platform and perform (sing, give a reading, etc.).

In still later years there was "formal" initiation, which was quite different. Each big sister gave a charge to her little sister, lighted a candle for her, or gave her a rosebud. This ceremony was planned by the junior class, and all students and faculty attended. It was one of the highlights of training. Some very solemn commitments were made to the profession at these formal initiation services.

To keep control over the situation the faculty required class members to write up their entire plans for initiation—formal and informal—and present them one week prior to the event.

Doris said that one of the happiest memories of her training was the day when I took the whole first-year class to Kansas City on the Public Service Bus to get fitted with black duty shoes. An orthopedic surgeon had already examined the students' backs and feet and prescribed the proper make of shoe for each. Black shoes and stockings were worn with uniforms until 1943 because Miss Copeland felt that the girls would not keep white shoes, shoe laces, and hose clean.

After all the students were fitted with shoes they went on to the Forum Cafeteria for supper. Each girl was allowed to spend one dollar on the meal of her choice. After eating they went to a movie chosen by the majority.

Students were fitted with uniforms and given a week to break in their new shoes before *the day* arrived—the first day of duty on the hospital wards caring for real patients. The night before, most students couldn't sleep well for thinking they might forget everything they had learned in the nursing laboratory and while practicing procedures on each other. A few students would be so worried they would try to find reasons for leaving school.

After the girls had been introduced to their patients for the day by the instructor, most of them calmly took over and functioned as if they had been practicing nurses since the days of Florence Nightingale. It was an important milestone on the way to becoming RNs. Nearly all students felt it to be one of the most outstanding experiences in their lives.

After her graduation Doris Eliason married George Caster and became an industrial nurse for Hallmark in

Kansas City. She served there many years before her retirement. She then became active in the Nurses' Alumnae Association, serving as chairman of the publicity committee. She has taken art lessons and devotes much of her time to painting. Her work has been shown at art fairs and exhibits. She also has given some of her paintings to the Sanitarium.

As a member of the Hospital Auxiliary, Doris serves as a volunteer at the San, frequently at the information desk. She finds satisfaction in being among those persons who donate thousands of hours of free service so that care may be more satisfactory and less costly for the patients.

WILDA LEE HANSON WHILES

Wilda Lee Hanson came from Clarence, Missouri. A typical country girl, she was sturdy and had an appealing twinkle in her eyes. She was attuned to show merriment at the slightest provocation. Poor instructors who misspoke! She was certainly not unkind but if I said something in class that didn't come out exactly as I meant it to I could always depend on catching her eye and realize that she had picked up my faux pas.

She was well liked by everyone—students, patients, supervisors, instructors, and casual acquaintances. She had one major liability—her handwriting was atrocious. I remember telling her one day, "Wilda Lee, if I got a letter from Timbuktu in that handwriting I'd know it came from you."

She served in the Army Nurse Corps during World War II. One day I received a letter in that "famous" handwriting. The opening sentence was, "Miss Butterworth, I'm not in Timbuktu, but do you know who this letter is from? I'm in China." I was pleased to hear from her and know that she was doing good work in the Orient.

I can imagine that she made a wonderful nurse for sick and wounded soldiers. Her sense of humor would "save the day" in any hospital situation.

While she was in nursing school she had an acute attack of appendicitis and had to have an emergency appendectomy. She was given a spinal, and when the doctor put in the long needle to inject the anesthetic he must have touched a nerve because her left leg began to jerk. As usual her sense of humor came to the fore. She laughed and said, "I jerk just like the frog we 'pithed' in the anatomy laboratory." I hastened to reassure her that it would last just a few seconds and her fate would not be the same as that of the frog. She recuperated quickly from her operation and was soon back in class.

We lost track of her for a while after the war was over, then we learned that she was in the Veterans Hospital at Columbia, Missouri. She was being treated for cancer of the voice box. Several of her former instructors and classmates kept up a correspondence with her trying to encourage her and help her make the best of the life she had left. Finally we received a letter from a niece telling us of her death.

I feel sure that Wilda Lee is smilingly administering to the needs of people in the "land across the river Jordan." To be happy she'd have to be busy.

She had a good time in the School of Nursing. Her laugh was infectious, so she was a good influence on other students. That is why I am sure that wherever Wilda Lee is, she is being helpful in some capacity.

HELEN THORBURN BRICKER

Helen entered nursing school in the fall of 1939 at the same time as her cousin, Doris Eliason. Helen brought her widowed mother and a sister from Montana to Independence with her. Her father had been an RLDS minister. Helen was a good student and carried out all of her responsibilities as a nurse in a very creditable manner.

When I asked Helen to tell me some things she remembered that happened while she was in the school, she wrote the following:

1. Mother Thorpe rang the bell at 6:00 a.m. which seemed the middle of the night. In winter she would say, "Time to get up. It's a cold, dark day."

2. Mr. Mullins, one of my first patients, sent me cards, flowers, candy, and books every so often all the rest of his life (about ten years).

3. My first patient was almost as nervous as I when I first gave a bed bath. I bathed her and turned her just as we were taught, but she kept asking, "Please, won't you get me a nurse?"

4. "Aunt Emma," a patient in 109, was paralyzed on her whole left side. She was unable to talk except to say "da da da." She was there over the years for several classes to practice their skills and to become affectionately involved.

5. One night "Swede Hanson," another student nurse, took a nap and about 10:00 p.m. came tearing through my room ready to go to work. She thought she had slept all night.

6. While living at the Copeland House, 1413 West Truman Road, we were almost late every morning because the first one down had to

give Mother Copeland her insulin and it better be given correctly!

7. I particularly remember how Hospital Chaplain Almer Sheehy started our day with a peppy talk during Chapel (6:45-7:00 a.m.). This was the highlight of each day.

8. I shall be forever grateful to you, Miss Butterworth, for teaching us well and being so concerned as we adjusted to homesickness, a family crisis, and a new way of life.

After graduation Helen married Arthur Bricker. They have a daughter who is married and has a family of her own. Helen has been the evening supervisor at the San for many years where she is currently employed. A quiet person, she is respected for her nursing and administrative skills. She is also an active church member.

Helen's mother, Mrs. Victoria Thorburn, became a night housemother after the nurses' home was moved to the old Sanitarium building. She served faithfully in this capacity for many years.

The residence director, more commonly called housemother, was usually an older woman who had reared her family and still considered herself capable of "mothering" a big family of girls. Many student nurses were very fond of the housemothers and considered them close friends (and, if needed, advisers). Other students felt that the residence director was there only to see that the students obeyed school rules and regulations. They accused them of searching their rooms for contraband material, of waiting for them to come in late, of reading their letters. According to these students, nothing good came from anyone in authority.

At first a nurses' residence had only one director who lived in and was there twenty-four hours a day. As work schedules for other hospital personnel changed so did those of the residence directors. Eventually they worked a standard forty-hour week.

The housemothers I have been able to remember (who served for any length of time) have been Mrs. Sarah Thomas, Mrs. Mabel Thorpe, Mrs. Emma Beadnall, Mrs. Josephine Reese, Mrs. Victoria Thorburn, Mrs. Adeline Judd, Mrs. Williamson, Miss Grace Lovell, Mrs. Mary Copeland, Mrs. Mary Thomas, Mrs. Olive Draper Jones, Mrs. Vinnie Hatch, Mrs. Lulu Butler, Mrs. Mary Carter, Mrs. Gladys Duffey, Mrs. Mary Hunt, Mrs. Edith Lewis, Mrs. Ruth McNutt, and Mrs. Lola McQueen.

The 1957 *Sanilog* was dedicated to the housemothers as follows:

Because of your hours of service, your wealth of kindness, your ability to listen and help us live joyously, we the students wish to dedicate our 1957 *Sanilog* to you.

MARY LOU DENMAN STOBAUGH

Mary Lou Denman, of Michigan, first wrote to the San School of Nursing when she was in junior high school. (She always used white stationery with a flag sticker at the top.) She was sure she wanted to be a nurse and wrote to ask what subjects to take in high school to best prepare her for nursing school. At the completion of each year she would report her progress and ask which studies to select next year.

The day to enter training finally arrived in 1944. Mary Lou was a small bundle of energy with eyes twinkling and lips smiling. She was never too tired to do whatever needed to be done on duty, in the classroom, or as an extracurricular activity.

According to her records she worked in a spark plug factory's X-ray department (part of the emergency room). She wanted to be a nurse because she had seen such interesting things happen there. She had seen "a skull grow together" and "people get well."

She was in training during World War II when the school was sponsored and partially financed by the United States Cadet Nurse Corps. In the summer of 1942 I had gone to a nursing education workshop in LaSalle, Illinois, about ninety miles from Chicago. While we were there one of our speakers told us about the suggested U.S. Cadet Nurse Corps, set up by a law sponsored by Frances Payne Bolton, a Congresswoman from Ohio, and a friend to nursing. This speaker outlined its provisions, terms of application, and acceptance. When I came home I reported to Director Nelle Morgan, the school faculty, and the hospital Board of Directors. I was then invited to Research Hospital in Kansas City to explain what I knew about the U.S. Cadet Corps. Members of the hospital council and directors of schools of nursing attended. The upshot of this was that as soon as the bill passed, the San School of Nursing was ready to apply. I can remember praying, "Please help the San School of Nursing's application to the U.S. Cadet Corps to pass and I will work as hard as I can to make it a *good* school so that we can all feel proud of it." I did put forth much effort and, along with Nelle Morgan, tried to guide the school in ever improving channels.

During the Cadet Corps years enrollment increased to

101 students. Five classes were graduated (117 graduates). The Cadet Corps supplied summer outdoor uniforms of gray and white striped broadcloth with shoulder epaulets and gold buttons. The summer hat was gray with a red ribbon around it.

The winter uniforms were gray flannel with red epaulets, a gray felt tam that stood high in front and had a large cadet emblem. The students were asked to wear these whenever they were in public.

The Cadet Corps gave each student a stipend while she was in the school besides paying for all of her expenses—board, room, books, and tuition. At first the stipend was $15.00 a month; this was increased to $20.00 a month until the last six months when it became $30.00 a month.

Both the students and faculty decided that there should be military drills. The Missouri National Guard was asked to supply drill instructors and one evening a week the students drilled for from two to three hours. (Some of the nurses later married their drill officers.) These "exercises" promoted better posture and probably helped to make the students more physically fit. After the newness wore off, however, the drilling became a burden to some of the students.

During this time President Harry S Truman was in the White House. Consequently whenever the Trumans came to the Summer Whitehouse in Independence they were met with "pomp and circumstance." The students sometimes greeted them with armloads of roses for Mrs. Truman and Margaret. Some of the girls had their pictures taken with President Truman as he was being presented with a copy of the *Sanilog*. None of these "unofficial" photographs were permitted by the U.S. Government to be printed.

One day when the students were celebrating the Cadet Corps' birthday Mrs. Truman came to the tea given for them. She was most gracious and let the students snap pictures. (She kept the FBI out.)

We at the San School of Nursing will always have a warm spot in our hearts for this gracious first lady who did not think herself too good to be present for the occasion.

During the last six months in the School of Nursing the girls who wished to do so were allowed to work in a government hospital in some specialized nursing area. Quite a few took advantage of this opportunity. Their affiliations might be in medical, psychiatric, or surgical nursing.

When a student signed up with the U.S. Nurse Cadet Corps she had to promise to remain in government or essential nursing jobs for at least five years after completing her education.

Mary Lou married Kenneth Stobaugh, an RLDS missionary, and worked the 3:00 to 11:00 p.m. shift in a hospital near Nauvoo, Illinois, where her husband was in charge of church historical buildings and sites.

One night as she was coming home from work she was killed in an automobile accident. By this time her children were fairly well grown. Her warm personality, her cheerful smile, and "nursing know-how" are greatly missed. Wherever she is we know she is "about her Master's work."

IOLA TORDOFF

Iola came into the School of Nursing in September, 1944, after the U.S. Cadet Corps was functioning at the San. I often heard her say, "If it hadn't been for the Cadet Corps I could never have come in training. I could never have been a nurse."

After graduation from high school Iola was a legal secretary in Independence for seven years and an auditor for one year. When she attended Graceland (1943-44) she was older than most of the students in her class because she had had to work to save to attend college. As a student nurse she was mature, dependable, interested in the welfare of her patients and her fellow students.

She was also talented—a "whiz" at the typewriter, a vocal soloist, an artist, and a good church school teacher. When the School of Nursing had a contest to choose a bookplate Iola won first place. Thereafter thousands of library books were identifiable by the ISH School of Nursing Library Bookplate (a nurse seated at a table piled high with books, and looking at a world globe). As a student she was editor of the *Sanilog*; later she served as faculty sponsor for the yearbook.

After graduation from the San Iola did general staff nursing on the orthopedic floor for a year, then became an instructor of medical nursing.

In 1950-51 and 1954-55 she attended Western Reserve University and obtained her Bachelor's degree in Nursing. She then came back to the San and taught advanced medical-surgical nursing to the senior students. She took courses at the University of Kansas

City in the summers of 1955 and 1967, returned to Western Reserve University 1961-1963, and received her Master's degree in Medical-Surgical Nursing. Back at the San she became instructor in charge of clinical studies until August, 1967, when she went to work at the University of Kansas School of Nursing. Here she taught medical-surgical nursing and traveled to various areas of Kansas holding clinics and seminars on specific subjects so that nurses in the outlying areas of the state might have opportunity to learn the latest methods in nursing and keep updated as new nursing procedures and knowledge came to light. She was well fitted for such a role and became almost indispensable to the KU School of Nursing.

In 1969 she became associate professor of Graceland's Department of Nursing. Then she was hired as head of clinical studies at the San, which position she still holds.

Iola has served the church long and well in the health field. She has made a number of trips to Haiti with Health Teams, several times with student nurses.

The 1958 *Sanilog* was dedicated to her:

An architect of professional lives, a builder for the nurses of the future, a foundation for friendship, love and encouragement, a tool for our never ending search for learning.

Because you have so dedicated these qualities in our behalf, we joyously and gratefully dedicate this book to you, Miss Tordoff, and with it our warmest appreciation.

And, Miss Tordoff, we of the *Sanilog* Staff want to express an additional thanks for the fellowship we have enjoyed in working with you. You have certainly won a place in the heart of each of us. We realize your wonderful sponsorship has been responsible for all that went into this book of living memories. May you have His guidance always as you continue to walk in His ways.

JEAN NAGEL

Jean was a tall, slender, dark-eyed, dark-haired girl who smiled a lot. She did not appear to be a very forceful person but as we worked with her we learned differently. She was a combination of sweetness, earnestness, and firmness. Above all she had a genuine interest in people—especially in meeting the needs of those who were ill.

Before entering the School of Nursing in 1945 Jean worked for over a year as an aide at the San. She was a member of the Evangelical Church, which she attended regularly. Both in high school and at the San she was a good student; in state board exams she ranked first in her class.

After graduation Jean attended Moody Bible School in Chicago, then went to Ghana, Worawora, Togoland, in Africa as a missionary nurse. She spent half of her time doing missionary work and the other half giving nursing care. While at Worawora she worked in the operating room, in pharmacy, in central supply, in the outpatient department, and in teaching student nurses.

In 1968 Jean started working under the Sudan Interior Commission at Egbe, Nigeria, West Africa. For this assignment she studied Yoruba, the native language. In 1972 she started working at Oume on the Ivory Coast of West Africa. She has spent practically twenty-five years as a missionary nurse in Africa and apparently has enjoyed serving in that capacity.

Although her parents are deceased, Jean still has ties in Independence—relatives and her many friends at the Evangelical Church and the Sanitarium. She returns occasionally to rest, recuperate, study, and gain new professional skills.

Other San graduates have served in foreign lands under the auspices of some church. Those I know about include the following:

Dana Watts Ellis, Tahitian Islands
Elvina Richmond, Leprosy Colony, Philippine Islands
Iola Tordoff, Haiti
Jean Nagel, Gold and Ivory Coasts of Africa
Diana Worthington Guthrie, Philippine Islands
Rosalyn Green Coward, Laos
Marilyn Keiper Schaefer, Haiti
Therese "Tetua" Richmond, Tahiti
Elizabeth Jahn Smith, Honduras
Gail Beavers Coward, Honduras
Beverly Thompson McNutt, Honduras
Dana Ludy Watts, Africa
Laura Naylor Oppelt, Honduras
Joanne Sanner, Haiti
Dorcas Hentz Wilkinson, Ship *Hope* and Korea
Hoang Van Phi, Viet Nam
Doris Brooks Heath, Africa
Ava Wallace Gardner, Korea
Carol Propst Castillo, Honduras

There may be many more San grads who have worked in foreign lands, but these are the ones I personally know. All I have talked with have found the work to bring a kind of satisfaction obtained in few other nursing ventures. It requires use of their total faculties—education, nursing skills, ingenuity, and love. It also satisfies the natural desire for adventure and recognition.

Jean Nagel is spending her life satisfying not only

these desires but providing both spiritual and physical wholeness for some of the world's neediest people.

LILY NG MITSANAGA

When I hear the name Lily I think of a slender, fragile blonde with white skin and pale blue eyes. Lily Ng was just the opposite. A Polynesian from Hawaii, she was one of nearly fifty students from Hawaii who attended the San School of Nursing between 1941 and 1967.

Of average height, pleasingly plump, dark of skin, eye, and hair, Lily was an excellent student. The most striking thing about her was her ease of manner in all situations. She had an almost photographic memory, so learning came easy. Perhaps a few other students envied the apparent lack of effort with which Lily obtained A's on her tests and report cards.

Lily was a joy to her teachers. She was usually the last one to leave the classroom after class because she always had questions to ask so she could better understand her lessons and their application in caring for patients.

Since 1939 San students have had a three months affiliation at St. Louis State Hospital. Here Lily became "famous" because her name was the shortest on the roster of employees, students, and patients. Her last name, Ng (pronounced Ing), was so unusual that it even made the front page of a St. Louis newspaper.

After graduation Lily returned to St. Louis to work. While there she married, had a family, and worked as long as her health permitted. All too soon she died of cancer of the lung.

Another thing I will always remember about Lily and almost all other Hawaiians and Southerners were their reactions to the first snowfall each year. They would put on their wraps, dash gleefully out the door, lie down, roll in the snow, and throw handfuls at each other, laughing all the while.

They were soon taught by the Northerners how to build snow forts, make hard snowballs, and have snow battles. They made snowmen and snow women that stood long after the rest of the snow had melted. These warm-climate people were also very eager to go sleigh riding or sledding.

Back when I was a student nurse the police used to rope off Walnut Street from Lexington to Forrest so the boys and girls could have a good hill for their sleds. Many a student nurse went for such rides down Walnut Street with her boyfriend, town brother and sister, or another student nurse. But as Independence grew, the practice was discontinued.

Another winter treat—one that is still available—is snow ice cream. (Of course it should never be made from the first snowfall because that snow contains dirt that has collected in the air since the last snowfall.) The "recipe" calls for ½ teaspoonful of vanilla, sugar to taste, milk, and enough snow to make it the consistency of ice cream. I have enjoyed it ever since I was a small child. Whenever I see a layer of beautiful white snow on the ground, trees, and shrubbery, I not only remember my childhood experiences with snow but also recall the delight of the Hawaiian students. . . especially Lily.

EVELYN "FLOWERPOT" BERRYMAN BARRETT

Evelyn—better known as "Flowerpot"—Berryman entered the School of Nursing in September 1949 after receiving her A.A. degree from Graceland College.

Evelyn was a tall, slender girl who dressed according to her whim. I remember her in red plaid slacks waiting to practice for a variety show (this was in the days before many women wore slacks). She was creative, and in situations like a variety show she was tops both with her ideas and performance. We always knew Evelyn was around because she was original in anything she did. This was a good characteristic but occasionally had to be "guided."

I do not know where she went directly after graduation from the San in 1952, but I do know that she married Ward Leroy Barrett and a daughter, Kelli, was born to them. In 1956 Evelyn received her B.S. degree in Nursing from Ohio State University at Columbus; in 1962 she obtained her master's and in 1971 her Ph.D, also from Ohio State University. She majored in higher education administration with a minor in adult education. Her doctoral thesis was on Florence Nightingale and her contributions to hospitals, nursing, and nurses. I think the incentive to write on this subject may well have been triggered by her studies at the San.

Evelyn has been a staff nurse, an associate director of nursing service in a five-hundred-bed hospital, an associate executive director and counselor for the Ohio State Nurses' Association, and dean of nursing at Capitol University in Columbus, Ohio. At present she is dean of nursing at the University of Iowa in Iowa City. (I understand a Ph.D. course in nursing is soon to be offered there.) As far as I know Evelyn is the only San graduate who has completed work for a Ph.D. Her biography appears in *Who's Who of American Women* and *Who's Who in the Midwest.* She belongs to the American Nurses' Association, the National League of Nursing, and the American College and University Administrators.

Evelyn has been popular as a speaker and has been asked to speak at the San and Graceland on various special occasions. She has come far and been highly successful in spite of the fact that she entered nursing because of "the glamour of the uniform." She says she will never regret taking nurses' training.

I have great respect for her ability and accomplishments. From her I have learned some valuable lessons that are not presented in books. She jarred me from my complacency and made me think. I hope she can always keep this "spirit of rebellion" that leads to greater things.

The San School of Nursing was visited in 1951 by a consultant from the National League of Nursing and as I remember it was classified in the "B" group. Temporary accreditation was made so that the faculties of schools could learn their proper role in the School of Nursing—that of determining what student nurses needed to learn and how best to help them learn it.

The three major problems confronting schools of nursing at that time were long-standing problems:

a. Lack of prepared faculty.
b. Expense to the hospital of maintaining the school (it markedly affected patient care costs).

c. Service demands for the students' time that had to be fulfilled before educational demands could be met.

With the help of the consultant the school could be evaluated as to what was good or bad about it. The faculty was helped to see the value of the school's philosophy being formulated by group study, discussion, and agreement. This was used as a basis for organizing the educational program consisting of subject-matter classes in which repetition in different classes was eliminated and in which clinical supervision and teaching on the hospital ward helped to emphasize the students' knowledge of and skill in nursing care.

As more nurses became properly prepared to teach, the costs went up.

The San School of Nursing was visited in 1957 for full accreditation by two national nurse accrediting representatives. Their visit accomplished three purposes:

1. The out of state representative assisted in the evaluation of an out of state school of nursing.
2. She assisted in the evaluation of a school similar to the one where she was employed.
3. She learned better techniques in evaluating her own school or schools more realistically and impartially.

I acted as a second member of an accrediting team for diploma schools in three places: Temple, Texas; Wichita, Kansas; and Milwaukee, Wisconsin. Each time I had a different co-inspector.

The San School of Nursing received permanent accreditation in 1957, but some changes had to be made in the program before February, 1958, when it was rechecked by an NNAS accrediting team. Accreditation was retained from then until the close of the school in 1971. Never again were the accrediting team's consultants so feared. Actually working on our school self-evaluation and visits of an accrediting team became a relaxed, enjoyable co-adventure between faculty and the consultants.

In 1965 the American Nurses' Association came out with a position paper stating that "education for those who work in nursing should take the general system of education" (colleges, universities, etc.).

In 1966 the San received a government grant which permitted the hiring of Margaret McKevit, R.N., B.S., M.A., to do her study of the future of the school of nursing which eventually led to the closing of the diploma program and the establishing of the Graceland College program. The last San School of Nursing class was graduated in May 1971. The Graceland program has developed very rapidly, so that in recent years between forty and fifty students have been graduated annually.

Evelyn Berryman Barrett and Margaret McKevit have also been involved in the Nursing School Accreditation of College Schools of Nursing.

DORIS BECKSTROM

Doris was a "Salvation Army lassie" married to the commander of the Independence Post. She applied to enter the school in the fall of 1949 so she could become a nurse and assist her husband, who planned to go to Africa as a missionary. Doris was the first married woman to enter the School of Nursing. (I think the San was the first in the Kansas City area to allow this, just as it was the first school to permit students to marry and remain to complete their training.)

Doris was an excellent student, despite the fact that she had Salvation Army duties to carry out each day after she left school. She was tremendously motivated and enthusiastic in what she was doing; had she not been she could never have accomplished all she did in her three years in nursing school. I am sure that "God helps those who help themselves," especially when their life plan is to work for him after proper preparation. Doris was such a person.

Once when I had her in for "grade card conference" she told me of a traumatic experience she had had on the Square in Independence just before Christmas. It seems that each night as the Salvation Army bell ringers went off duty at their "kettle posts" around the Square, Doris was assigned to gather up the contributions and put them in a safe place. This one night it was late, dark, and the streets were slippery. As she crossed the intersection her feet slipped from under her and she fell headlong, spilling the contents of the kettle she carried. Coins rolled in all directions. She got up and, maintaining her composure, went about picking up the coins and returning them to the kettle. She didn't look around to see who might have observed her embarrassing moment; she merely completed her task as quickly as possible and went on her way. That was Doris! Inside she was probably laughing because she could always see the funny side of things, even when the joke was on her.

Doris was graduated in 1952. Soon after that she and her husband were sent to the Gold Coast in Africa.

Then in 1974 we received a long letter from Doris with a request for a copy of her nursing record so she could become licensed as an R.N. in a new area. At that time her oldest daughter was twenty-one, a graduate of Western Michigan University with a major in business home economics. Her nineteen-year-old daughter was attending North Michigan University and majoring in social service. Her fifteen-year-old daughter planned her future in the field of genetics, and her fourteen-year-old son wanted to build bridges. Doris planned to go to work at the veterans' hospital. Her husband had died in March of 1974, after being ill with Hodgkin's Disease for eight years.

In the 1950s we initiated a program called "Community and Social Health Aspects of Nursing." It was intended to familiarize the students with community health and social resources. Supposedly, if the students were familiar with these agencies in Independence, they could go into any community and learn the health resources there. The students were given a few classes at the beginning of the course, then went on field trips, wrote a report of each agency visited, and had class discussions once a week.

They seemed to enjoy these trips and learned a lot from them. Many of them investigated the agencies in their hometowns when they were home on vacation.

We felt this gave the students insight into the health field and helped them learn quickly that the hospital was not the only health agency or institution, but one of many. They also learned that in order to carry out a program of positive health and disease prevention in any community many other agencies were needed. The students became quite learned in this area and developed a wide interest in how they as citizens could promote such worthy causes.

Many San graduates have been active in church and other community activities, aside from their regular jobs. I like to think that they were motivated to participate because of this class and the field trips.

Doris Beckstrom gave much to the world community in the field of health, not only in the United States but in Africa.

CAROLYN JONES TAYLOR

Carolyn was one of the students who spent a year at Graceland prior to entering the San School of Nursing in September 1949. That year a greater number than usual of the students had attended Graceland. This meant that in 1952 they would graduate from Graceland with an A.A. degree; as soon as they passed state board exams, they would also have their R.N.'s.

Students were first registered in the state of Missouri about 1921. Anyone who had graduated before that date could pay the fee and become registered without taking the exams. Not every San graduate received this message, so in later years if they wished to become R.N.'s they had to take and pass the Missouri state board exams. Some were bitter about not receiving the notice (they had difficulty in recognizing that the fault was theirs for not keeping the school informed as to their current address).

While at the San Carolyn was an "A" student. She was active in the student-faculty organization and extracurricular activities such as variety shows, yearbook, newspaper, and sports.

One of the areas in which various students helped the school administration was recruitment. Later, as graduates, they helped with "San Day" services to raise finances for the School of Nursing.

After I became a full-time instructor the fall of 1935 we published our first school of nursing catalog. After that a new one was published every two or three years so that prospective students would have up-to-date information on entrance requirements, school facilities, and the nursing program. The first two catalogs did not contain pictures, but after that they featured photographs of students in the classrooms, on ward duty, and in extracurricular activities.

In the forties, fifties, and sixties we usually had several recruitment brochures published every year or so. Frequently we took programs to Graceland College to promote San recruitment among the students there. I remember one year we role-played the teaching of a diabetic patient. Another year, after World War II, Dorothy Scholl told of her experiences as an army nurse and prisoner of war. We usually took large posters to display prominently around the college, and the students in uniform talked informally with students about health careers. They were fairly successful in their recruitment.

We also recruited in local and nearby high schools.

Sometimes we had representatives at junior high school "Career Days." At other times programs were presented by graduate nurses and students in assemblies or vocational classes. Occasionally some of our students and graduates participated in radio and television programs in a city-wide nurse recruitment program.

For a number of years the student nurses held a tea at the Nurses Home for high school girls interested in nursing. The guests were then taken on a tour of the Nurses Home and hospital.

The first San School of Nursing Day, sponsored by the church in all branches, was held in 1949. Money taken in at the collection not earmarked for some other purpose came to the San School of Nursing for use in upgrading the nursing program.

Publicity for San Day began early in the year with a letter from the First Presidency asking members to participate in the offering. Each month thereafter an article about the San and the School of Nursing appeared in the *Herald*. The write-up was usually accompanied by photographs. Before San Day each pastor was mailed literature with sermon suggestions for that day. Graduates of the School of Nursing were also sent this same packet of material and asked to participate in the service at their church.

This created much interest in the School of Nursing and aided greatly in the recruitment program. Many prospective students visited the San while in Independence to attend World Conference. In later years the recruitment of students for the diploma program at the San was dropped. Many students wanted a Bachelor's degree in Nursing without having to spend six years getting it. It was much easier to take a four-year college nursing course. So in the spring of 1971 the San School of Nursing graduated its last class and Graceland College graduated its first nursing class.

Carolyn Jones married Chester Taylor. They moved to the West Coast and had a family. Not long after graduation Carolyn went to Avila College in Kansas City where she received her bachelor's degree. Since then she has received her master's from the University of Oregon. Dr. Evelyn Berryman Barrett gave the commencement address at her former classmate's graduation.

San School of Nursing graduates have made and continue to make a significant contribution to the nursing profession and the world health program.

LOIS BROWNE DIMMIT and MARTHA SMITH HAMLINE

Lois came from Springfield, Missouri, in September 1949 to enter the School of Nursing. She was a tall blonde with a contagious smile and twinkling blue eyes. Her best friend was Martha Smith, a dark-haired, dark-eyed, heavy-set girl whose policeman father was killed in the Union Station Massacre June 14, 1928, when she was only four months old. While attending high school Martha worked part time at the Wee Wisdom Home Nursery and the Friendly Corner Drugstore.

Both Lois and Martha were involved in practically every extracurricular activity sponsored by the student nurses. Besides that, both were excellent students and made good grades on the National League of Nursing Achievement Tests and state board examinations. Martha had a glorious voice; she sang in a church choir, at chapel services, and religious emphasis programs, as well as at variety shows and hospital programs. Sometimes Lois and Martha sang duets.

Lois married Mr. Dimmit, editor of the newspaper at Wentzville, Missouri, (near St. Louis). She stayed at home to rear her family. As far as I know she did not pursue her nursing career. Martha married Mr. Hamline and also had a family. She became a medical supervisor at the San.

LUCILLE GRESS

Lucille was older than most girls when she came to the School of Nursing in 1951. She had not graduated from high school because she had to work to support her younger brothers and sisters. Later she took the G.E.D. Test and received credit for high school graduation. Lucille was very determined to learn everything that would help her to be a better nurse. She stayed after class to ask questions and probe the teacher's mind. Occasionally she would appear in the educational director's office to find out how she was doing grade wise and to offer soft-voiced suggestions. She was quiet but not timid. She spoke up if she had anything to say (and she usually did have) but she always did this in a calm voice.

Lucille made the highest grades in her class. After

graduation she attended the University of Kansas City and received her bachelor's and master's degrees in 1962 and 1966. After being graduated with honors, she taught surgical nursing at the San.

In September 1966 she became a faculty member at the University of Kansas School of Nursing where she still teaches.

Lucille has great respect for professional standards. She also has great concern for the welfare of her students and their patients. She can provide inspired leadership when it is needed, but she also can be an understanding follower. Lucille was active in the RLDS Professional Nurses' Association.

Lucille has made good progress in her professional life at the KU Medical Center School of Nursing and in the state of Kansas where she has conducted workshops and seminars for nurses in rural areas.

MARGARET McKEVIT

Margaret's mother Mabel Andrews, was a 1931 graduate of the San. Margaret, an only child, was beautiful, intelligent, and well liked. She was always an optimist and gave the impression that there was nothing that could not be done if one made up one's mind.

Before entering the San School of Nursing she had done some secretarial work for the church, some modeling, and some bookkeeping at a children's hospital in Canada. While attending Graceland she worked in the college library.

At the San she was a good student, interested in extracurricular activities (acting, school yearbook, art decorations, handcraft, tennis) and liked meeting and working with people. Her ambition was to get a degree. I can still remember her in a "cancan" lineup at a dinner that was given at the end of the nutrition course to test the students' ability to cook—and to furnish entertainment. Members of the hospital board of directors and their wives were invited. I think that the "cancan" bit was supposed to shock some of the guests. I must say that the girls did a good imitation of the real thing.

Margaret was popular with both sexes. She had the ability to discuss intelligently any subject that came up, but she never belittled the knowledge of others.

After graduation from the San she served as a staff nurse and night supervisor. Margaret wanted further education, however, so after working for a while she attended the University of Colorado where she obtained her Bachelor's degree in Nursing in 1958.

After that she went to New Orleans where she taught communicable disease nursing at the old and famous Charity Hospital founded in the 1700s. After three years there she returned to Colorado University to get her Master's degree in Nursing Education Administration (1962). She stayed on at the university to receive her specialist rating in maternal-child health nursing. Then she went to the University of Wisconsin where she taught from 1963 to 1966.

She came back to Independence to conduct a study of the San School of Nursing under a grant from the U.S. Department of Health and Welfare. This took from July 1, 1966, until the study's publication in August of 1967. It was titled "Exploration for Curriculum Revision."

Many people were involved in this study—students, instructors, directors, supervisors, head nurses, auxiliary personnel, physicians, members of the Board of Directors, Alumnae Association officers and members, School of Nursing Advisory Committee, hospital administrators, nurses employed by representative public health agencies, and representatives of hospitals in which San students went on affiliation. Working committees were formed from these various groups.

The study of the existing program included an evaluation of recruitment, admissions, and attrition rates; faculty and faculty organization; curriculum; extracurricular activities; library; services of students; physical facilities such as classrooms, clinical areas, and living conditions; and financial support. The final area was the evaluation of all data in terms of strengthening the diploma program and determining the future pattern of nursing education to be offered by, or in conjunction with, a college or university. Areas for special studies included students enrolled in the current program, alumnae members of this nursing program, admission policies and attrition rates, and limited college credit transferable to the N.L.N. accredited baccalaureate nursing program.

In 1965 Graceland had appointed a committee to make a "Report of the Campus Extension Committee." This "feasability study" was made with the supposition that the second Graceland Campus would be located in Independence for the Collegiate Nursing Program. The World Conference turned down the idea of the second Graceland Campus.

After the extensive study of the "Exploration for Curriculum Revision" published in August, 1966, however, Margaret McKevit was appointed Director of Nursing Studies at Graceland College in 1967. She immediately formed a committee for beginning organization of a Graceland Collegiate Nursing Program. The student nurses would remain on the Graceland Campus for the first two years, then obtain their clinical practice in Independence, Kansas City, and Liberty, Missouri, the last two years, graduating with a Bachelor of Science in Nursing.

Since the curriculum would be taught partly in Iowa and partly in Missouri the school had to be approved by both the Iowa and Missouri state boards of nursing. Consultation with members of the National Nurse Accrediting Agency helped Graceland planners formulate a sound degree nursing program.

The number of students being graduated from the Graceland Nursing Program has grown steadily throughout its eight years of existence.

1971-13	1975-46
1972-15	1976-51
1973-22	1977-39
1974-24	1978-40

Margaret McKevit took a year's leave of absence from 1975 to 1976 to rest, regain her health, attend seminars, and inspect collegiate nursing schools for the accrediting service. She then resigned as professor of the Department of Nursing at Graceland and accepted a position in the Department of Nursing at Louisiana University in New Orleans.

When I asked about her resignation she replied, "I'm not saying that I'll never come back to Graceland, but I do feel the need of getting experience in other institutions."

HOANG VAN PHI

She told us to call her "Phi," but whether that was her first or last name I didn't know. She explained very precisely how names are used in her country, but I didn't understand what she was saying. (Phi spoke native Vietnamese translated into English by way of French.)

Her brother-in-law was in some type of diplomatic service in Washington, and Phi attended American University there to become more proficient in English. She was sent to our school in 1953 by Margaret Willhoit from St. Luke's Hospital in Kansas City. Margaret was a friend of Nelle Morgan, Shirley Butler, and several San graduates who had worked with her in Missouri District No. 2 Nurses' Association. At that time she was with the U.S. Public Health Service in Washington in charge of foreign students coming to the States to study nursing under the auspices of the U.S. government. Margaret had picked our school of nursing for Phi because it was relatively small and everyone at the hospital was concerned about the welfare of the students. Phi, she felt, would get her share of loving attention and as much personal help as she needed.

Phi had Mabel McKevit as her town mother. Mabel proved to be a real mother to Phi, helping her select appropriate American clothes and making her feel welcome in her home at any time she was off duty. Phi was tiny, with coal black hair and eyes and a smile that spread clear across her face. She took a very active part in all school activities, often appearing in her native dress.

After graduation in 1958 she went back to Vietnam and worked for the government in a big Saigon hospital. She wrote nursing procedure books in Vietnamese and taught both male and female student nurses. Whenever there was a different case in the hospital Phi was called upon to organize the proper nursing care and tell others how to carry it out. She did exceptionally fine work, but her government did not see fit to pay her. She had very elderly grandparents and her own parents to help.

When the ship *Hope* went to Vietnam so its "crew" could teach the natives advanced nursing and other professional techniques Phi was there to serve as interpreter. Some of her friends in the States saw her picture with the *Hope* personnel on a newsreel at a local theater. She stayed with the ship as long as it docked at a Vietnamese port.

Sometime later Phi came back to the United States and attended college at Wayne University but was called home before the year was up due to some official misunderstanding between the U.S. and Vietnamese diplomats.

Throughout the years Phi has kept up a correspondence with many of her U.S. friends. I have always been pleased to get her quaint Vietnamese Christmas cards and hear how she is doing. She finally gave up hope of ever receiving pay from her government for her nursing services, so she resigned and started to work for the U.S. Embassy in Saigon.

As the Americans withdrew troups from Vietnam, they also began to transport the natives out of the country. Phi's aged grandparents elected to live out their lives in Vietnam and Phi stayed until the last plane (her parents came to the States ahead of her). She continued her nursing in every refugee camp she came to. She wanted to get as many out as possible.

Late in 1975 Phi came to her sister's home in California. Most of their belongings had been lost, but they were happy to escape alive. Phi would have to start over again to study for the licensing exam before she could practice as a registered nurse in California. A number of her Independence friends sent her money to help supplement her income.

Phi went to college in California while she was working and recently passed the LPN exam. She is continuing her college work in the hope that eventually she will be able to become a registered nurse. I hope that the prayers of her many friends will bring her in triumph through this time of trial.

Other San employees and graduates served during the Vietnam War. Jean Clark, a former instructor at the San, helped to care for wounded and ill soldiers being air transported from Vietnam to U.S. government hospitals. Georgia Shaw, a San graduate, spent time nursing in army hospitals in Vietnam.

I always have been proud of the way San girls have fulfilled their missions and conducted themselves professionally in whatever situation they have found themselves.

SHIRLEY HAYWARD PHILLIPS

Shirley transferred to the San School of Nursing in 1956 after attending Missouri Methodist Hospital School of Nursing at St. Joseph for two years. Prior to that she had been a telephone operator. Shirley says she went into nursing because she liked to help people with problems. She wanted to work under the auspices of the RLDS Church by helping the Saints and humanity in general physically, mentally, and spiritually.

In order to finish her nursing education at the San she had to sacrifice one year of her previous schooling since we had a ruling that no student could graduate without spending two calendar years in the San curriculum. Shirley complied and was graduated on August 27, 1958. Before graduation, however, she married Jerry Phillips. They lived in Independence and both worked. When their first baby was born dead they were broken-hearted until the birth of their daughter Lynda. A few years later they had a son, Gary. Both Shirley and Jerry devoted much time in meeting the needs of their two growing children.

Once, while on a picnic at Lake Jacomo, Shirley was bitten by a copperhead and taken to Jackson County Hospital for treatment. In the meantime her husband called the chaplain at the Sanitarium to come to administer to her, which he did. He also called their church prayer circle to start praying for her.

Shirley was seriously ill for two days but gradually improved and was permitted to go home. This proved to be a real spiritual experience both for her and for the family.

In 1971 Shirley and I worked with John Macek, coordinator at the Northeastern Jackson County Mental Health Center and the occupational therapist from Western Missouri Mental Health Center, to set up a day care center for the emotionally disturbed patients who came to the center for treatment. The patients were seen by a psychiatrist or social worker and assigned to the center for treatment. We maintained a varied program of handcrafts, games, ceramics, artwork, creative writing, and drama. It was gratifying to see the behavioral improvement in patients after two or three sessions at the center.

Shirley and I not only planned the programs but carried them out, buying the necessary supplies, reporting to the patients' doctors and getting them to suggest activities suitable to the needs of each individual.

The center was housed in the building that had been the nurses' dormitory. The whole first floor was used in one capacity or another. The crew was composed largely of volunteers unacquainted with a mental health program. Shirley worked there for over a year, and I spent four years at the center.

Dr. G. Leonard Harrington was medical superintendent of the Sanitarium in the early twenties. Later he specialized in psychiatry and for a number of years lectured in psychiatry at a Kansas City school of nursing. All senior students in the Kansas City area, including those of the San, attended these lectures. Our girls, however, had no actual contact with psychiatric patients until we arranged a three months' affiliation in psychiatric nursing at the St. Louis City Sanitarium. This experience was first offered to San students graduating in 1939. Even then it was not a mandatory part of the curriculum, as students were permitted to choose either psychiatric nursing in St. Louis or public health nursing with the Kansas City Visiting Nurse Association. Later the Board of Nursing made the psychiatric experience mandatory for all diploma nursing programs.

At the time when psychiatrists were few, most emotionally disturbed people were guided only by their family physicians. When I first encountered psychiatric patients I was both intrigued and frightened.

I remember that while still a probie I was on night duty for a month on second floor. One evening after the older student nurse working with me had gone to bed for her three hours off duty, I heard a strange noise on the stairway between the first and second floors. When I went to investigate I discovered a tall, distinguished looking man wearing nothing but a hat, a necktie, and shoes. I was startled until I realized that poor Mr. H. had somehow escaped his locked room. I promptly returned him to the nurse on first floor. (He was suffering from bromide poisoning, having imbibed too freely of this sleep-producing soporific.)

Another patient, Floyd B., was eighteen or twenty years old. I don't remember the exact diagnosis of his condition, but I do remember some of his pet sayings. He went around wrapped Indian fashion in a white bath blanket, and whenever he met anyone in the halls (which he paced continuously) he would throw open his blanket, extend his arms, and cry, "I'm a man and proud of it!" Another frequent expression of his (when anyone tried to give him a hypodermic injection) was, "I don't want a hippo, a flippo, or any other kind of o."

Women also had mental disturbances. Georgiana was a little old lady in her seventies or eighties who wore pigtails on each side of her head. In her prime she had been a Twelfth and Cherry Street prostitute. She was thoroughly confused, and happy only when she sat in a rocking chair rocking her baby—a rolled-up bath blanket.

Another patient I remember was Evelyn, also a street-walker, who was brought in from a car accident bleeding from one ear. She became a raving maniac with superhuman strength. Once while I was on night duty I took her her bedtime dose of paraldehyde. She grabbed it out of my hands, swallowed it in one big gulp, and asked for a pint more of the same. I explained that that was all the doctor had ordered. She reached up, pinned my hands together at the wrists with one of hers, and with the other beat me over the head until I thought it would crack. I was badly frightened, not knowing any way to get help and being unable to break away from her. Suddenly I bent down and bit her on the wrist and when she jerked back I pulled away from her. Perhaps this was not ethical, but it *was* extremely effective!

Later Evelyn was moved down to first floor to a room supposedly cleared of all things that she might use to harm herself or others. Over the door (which was kept locked) was a glass transom. Evelyn got out of bed, removed the small drawer from the table in her room, pulled a chair over to the door and stood on it. She still couldn't reach the transom so she climbed up on the doorknob. Shattering the glass with the desk drawer, she very carefully removed the spicules of glass from the transom frame, and climbed—into the arms of waiting nurses and doctors.

The faculty felt that San students had worthwhile experiences at the affiliate hospital in St. Louis. They learned not only psychiatric nursing but also how to adjust to a new situation away from the home school. Many of them became very active in the RLDS church in St. Louis because they had difficulty adjusting to the "big city" and to psychiatric patients, new instructors, and living in a dormitory with students from other schools.

The St. Louis Saints were gracious to the San students. They took the girls to church, to social functions, and to their homes. Students usually either liked psychiatric nursing or they hated it. Dillie Rose Gulmi, one of their instructors, used to say, "San students cry when they come and cry when they go." They cried when they arrived because they were homesick and frightened. They cried when they left because they were leaving many friends among the personnel, patients, and Saints. Some returned to St. Louis after graduation and worked at the state hospital.

The Mental Health Center in the "old San" can finally offer full psychiatric services—outpatient department, inpatient hospitalization, emergency care, children's services, and day care center. Currently the outpatient department occupies floors one and two, and inpatient services occupy the second floor of the 1943 Sanitarium building. I understand that eventually Northeastern Jackson County Mental Health Center will construct another building elsewhere and the original Sanitarium completed in 1909 will be torn down.

Shirley Phillips was just one of the San graduates who helped provide care for mental patients in Independence and Eastern Jackson County.

BARBARA THOMAN CURTIS

Barbara was a very good nurse and made great growth strides while a student at the San. She ranked high in both clinical practice and classroom theory. While in school she was president of both the student body and the student council.

During her senior year (1960) she represented the San in the second district student nurse speech contest and won. Then as representative of the Second District of Missouri Nurses' Association, she also won the state contest. As "Miss Missouri Student Nurse" she was a candidate for the national contest held in Florida. That year Barbara set something of a record. She was graduated one night, married to Richard Curtis the next, and they combined honeymoon and participation in the National Student Nurse Convention.

Barbara and Richard had three children. They lived in Washington State where Barbara went to college, taught in schools of nursing, served as president of the Washington State Nurses' Association, and was "bargaining agent" for nurses in that state. As a result of her work in Washington she became an employee of the American Nurses' Association and now travels widely around the United States.

Barbara is intelligent, enthusiastic, knowledgeable, energetic, and ambitious. Although she has not been well physically for several years she lives a very full and productive life.

JOYCE RICHARDSON SHIREMAN

Joyce entered the San School of Nursing in September, 1959. Before that she worked as a clerk and a part-time librarian. She also attended Graceland for one year. In her home congregation she served as organist and music director.

Joyce liked to be around people and be of service to them. (She always helped get Christmas baskets ready for the poor.) Therefore, her choice of nursing for a career was a natural.

She was a very good student—dependable, cooperative, conscientious, and empathetic. She continued to use her musical ability in the school and was always willing to help with extracurricular activities (usually as a leader). She was active in the student organization first as a student and later as a faculty member.

Mrs. Bernice White and Joyce worked out classes and clinical experience for camp nursing. Students in the last few classes graduated from the San spent a week in camp nursing. This equipped them to serve more effectively as nurses at reunions and children, youth, and specialized camps (diabetic, cerebral palsy, cystic fibrosis, geriatric, etc.). The original camp nursing manual written by Dorothy Hays, R.N. (1948), was modeled after the *National Camping Manual.*

Joyce taught medical-surgical nursing at the San before becoming Mrs. Shireman. She and her husband have one son. Joyce studied at the University of Iowa, the University of Kansas Medical Center, and received her master's degree from Ohio State University at Columbus. Since the family has moved to Ohio she has been teaching nursing there.

In 1977 she rewrote the Camp Health Supervision manual, and it was published for the RLDS Professional Nurses' Association.

BEVERLY THOMPSON NUTT

Beverly Thompson, from Yukon Territory in Canada, was one of the bravest student nurses I have ever known. Her family lived a relatively isolated life in a cold and snowy land. Beverly graduated from high school in a class of one. Although she had little competition she was far from a mediocre student. She could hold her own with the most brilliant students in class.

Beverly was a quiet, cheerful member of any group. Although she usually had little to say, she had a merry twinkle in her eyes. While she was in the School of Nursing her mother entered a Canadian hospital and was told that she had terminal cancer. Beverly offered to go home and care for her mother, but her mother insisted that she stay and complete her nursing education. She stayed—and gave it all she had.

Everyone was feeling sorry for her on the day her

mother died, but Beverly did not indulge in self-pity. She was doing what her mother had wanted her to do. There are many forms of courage. Beverly had her own particular brand.

Shortly after completing her nursing course, Beverly Thompson and a classmate, Gail Beavers (Coward), went to Honduras for a year at La Buena Fe Clinic, providing health care in an area where no other medical facilities existed. Under the pressure of work and living among Spanish-speaking people they picked up the language very quickly.

Beverly is married to David Nutt, R.N., and lives in Calgary, Alberta, Canada, where she is an instructor of aides and orderlies in the Foothills Hospital. She and her husband have a son and a daughter.

Beverly was a student who enjoyed all of her nursing experiences.

MARY JO MADER KITTINGER

After two years at Graceland, two years of work, marriage, and three children, Mary Jo was older and more mature than the other members of her class. She had been a bookkeeper and executive secretary, and—at church—a choir director and organist. Although her life was already full, she decided she wanted a service career that would let her express her love of people. Her family agreed and were most cooperative in helping to make arrangements so that she might be able to attend the San School of Nursing.

From the time she began her nursing education, Mary Jo was always at the head of her class. She made straight "A's" all through school. She was always up-to-date on the latest nursing methods. While a student she attended almost all of the extracurricular activities and usually brought her children with her.

After graduation she worked in the operating room at the San and became operating room clinical instructor in the school. She completed work for her bachelor's degree at Central Missouri State University at Warrensburg. Her students respected her because she was always enthusiastic and worked well under stress.

When I was in training students spent five and a half months in the operating room. While there they made hospital supplies—dressings, cotton applicators, cotton balls, sponges for operations—and learned to run the autoclave (the sterilizer would be full of surgical dressings, operation packs, drums, sterile solutions, and instruments). Students also learned to "roust" for first minor operations; that is, they were to wait on the "scrubbed" nurse and doctors—give them sterile supplies, tie the doctor's and scrub nurse's gowns, and count sponges used.

Later in their o.r. instruction the students learned to scrub for minor operations (tonsillectomies, nose operations, rectal and vaginal surgery). Still later they did first and second scrubs for major operations (abdominal, Caesarian, pelvic, gall bladder, amputations, brain and bone surgery). Each student had to scrub for a certain number of major and minor operations to get credit for her o.r. experience. When I was a student, nurses in o.r. also scrubbed for the delivery of babies. I enjoyed this experience very much. It made me feel necessary and proficient.

Later the student nurses who were on obstetric service rather than o.r. nurses were "on call" for the delivery of babies. This was better because they had the opportunity to see the patient before delivery, immediately after, and for the next five days. They also had the opportunity to care for the baby and get the mother and baby ready to go home—physically, mentally, and emotionally. This was considered "total patient care."

Mary Jo taught o.r. clinical nursing until the school was closed June 1, 1971. At present she is working as assistant to a neurosurgeon. As is her life's pattern, she is doing well in that capacity.

KATHLEEN MURPHY REVELL

Kathy came into the School of Nursing in September 1966. She studied diligently, took good care of her patients, and participated enthusiastically in extracurricular activities. Her sunny smile and sparkling eyes made her a joy to her instructors. (I don't mean by that that she didn't stand up for what she thought was right even though it might be contrary to our viewpoint. She could argue logically, yet leave us without rancor if she came out ahead.)

After graduation she enrolled at Graceland College and received a B.S. degree in nursing in 1972. There she made the dean's list and received the Nelle Morgan Leadership Award. She served one term as president of the RLDS Professional Nurses, then married Roger

Revell who works for the music department of the world church. They have a son, Andy, and a daughter, Amy. Kathy is now working full time at the Northeastern Jackson County Mental Health Center.

Kathy had no relatives in Independence but enjoyed the relationship with her town family and her "big sister," Stella Oleksy Bird, who was a year ahead of her in training.

Kathy arrived at the Nurses' Home a day earlier than the rest of the new students and was met at the house-mother's desk by her big sister who took her to her room, helped her unpack, and introduced her to the local shopping area.

From the time that I entered training each new student had a junior for a "big sister." After she finished her freshman year she was assigned a senior big sister, and she herself was given a little sister to guide.

A "big sister" greeted her charge upon her arrival and saw that she was properly initiated, telling her how to get off on the right foot with the other older students, instructors, and supervisors. She coached the newcomer in hospital ethics, showed her how to wear her uniform properly, and often introduced her to new boyfriends. She acted as a counselor whenever little sister was in trouble, was discouraged, sick, or lonely. She also acted as a "sounding board." In fact big and little sisters often shared their common successes, failures, positive and negative emotions. They supported or comforted each other as the occasion warranted. Most of them became fast friends and kept in touch for the remainder of their lives.

DANA LUDY WATTS

Dana entered the School of Nursing in September 1966 at the age of nineteen. She had attended Graceland College and while there worked in the Graceland Infirmary. During high school she was a nurse aide in the county hospital. She put on her application that she wanted to become a visiting nurse and later to work in Mexico.

Dana was a tiny girl with big brown eyes and brown hair. She was intelligent; during her three years in the school she made a straight "A" average and ranked first in her class of forty-three. Although she was small, she always did her share. She was also a high achiever. One of her sources of inspiration was the convocation program.

In the 1960s faculty members decided that the students' education and viewpoints might be too narrowly focused on health, nursing, and hospital life. To foster a broader interest, convocations were instituted. They were held once a month, and everyone who could attend was urged to do so.

A committee consisting of representatives from various groups planned the programs and made all arrangements including publicity. There was a variety of subject matter and a variety of speakers.

The convocations were usually well attended. They were a highlight in the school program for the students.

Dana and her husband are living in Africa at the present time. It's not *Mexico*, but it is a foreign land.

LAUREL OPPELT

Laurel attended Graceland in 1941. Then she was married and had two sons. After she and her husband were divorced she felt divinely directed to prepare herself as a nurse. Being RLDS she wanted to obtain her nursing education at the San. She entered in September 1967, leaving her grown son in Washington State and bringing her younger with her to Independence. They rented an apartment near the high school and only several blocks from the hospital.

Laurel was an intelligent, aggressive, studious person. While in the School of Nursing she was usually chairman or a member of the worship committee and worked with the chaplain to plan the student's religious activities.

Laurel had long felt that she would like to serve in some Spanish-speaking country. This desire was fulfilled when she went to Honduras as a missionary nurse. We hear good reports of her work there as well as in the state of Washington.

VIDA BUTTERWORTH

This personality sketch will be more complete than the others because I have more information about the subject.

I realize that I could have achieved little without the help of my heavenly Father, my parents, relatives, and the people at the Sanitarium and School of Nursing with whom I associated.

I was born in Dow City, Iowa, on Thanksgiving morning November 30, 1905. (I'm told Mom had the dinner cooked and ready for all the rest of the family.) I attended school in Dow City, graduating from high school in 1924. I then taught rural school for two years before entering training at the San June 1, 1926. I was graduated on July 31, 1929.

For two years I worked as a private duty nurse and then joined the hospital staff as night nurse on the obstetric floor and as assistant night supervisor from 1931 to 1933. I attended the nursing department of Teacher's College, Columbia University, New York, the summers of 1931 and 1932 preparing myself to be an instructor of nursing.

In 1933-34 I served as college nurse at Graceland, at the same time attending the college as a student. At the end of that school year I obtained an Associate of Science degree. I never did get to attend a football game on Saturday as that was the time I did most of my studying (students were seldom ill enough on Saturday to require the nursing services).

I was required to take physical ed and became proficient at chasing tennis balls, setting up bowling pins, etc. I remember a gym show while I was there in which eight of us tap-danced to "The Sidewalks of New York." I was very sincere about my tap-dancing but I was awkward. I can laugh about it now. Although I no longer tap I do interpretive dancing to records in the secrecy of my living room. It's good for my muscles and digestion.

I attended Teachers College at Columbia University again in 1934-35 and received my Bachelor of Science in Nursing Education. I returned to Independence and began teaching in the School of Nursing in August 1935. There I taught until the closing of the school in June 1971.

I received my Master of Arts degree from Columbia University in June 1941. I belonged to the RLDS Professional Teachers Association and am still a member of the RLDS Professional Nurses' Association. I also belonged to the San Nurses' Alumnae, Second District Nurses' Association, the American Nurses' Association, and the local, state, and national League for Nursing. I served as officer, chairperson, and/or committee member for all of these organizations except the national ones. I was chairman of the Kansas City Educational Directors of Schools of Nursing and was on the editorial board of *Missouri's Nurses* in 1957.

Students dedicated the *Sanilog* to me in 1950-51 and in 1962. The dedicatory comments were as follows.

Miss Vida Butterworth, R.N., B.S., M.A., Educational Director of the Independence Sanitarium and Hospital School of Nursing, is known for her patience in the classroom, her understanding of human behavior, her wisdom in social and educational situations, and her will to follow and to lead. She has given of her time and talents for the molding of young women into mature, capable, and alert nurses and citizens. In appreciation of Miss Butterworth do we respectfully dedicate this 1950-51 *Sanilog.*

Like a tree with leaves outspread
To shelter all who come below,
Like a tree, of you it's said,
The passing years have watched you grow.

As we stand here in your shade
And take the knowledge that you give,
Our lives are finer, richer made,
Inspired by the life you live.

Tree roots, mighty and unseen,
Are like your spirit, great and true.
Like spring leaves so fresh and green,
You bring new life to all you do.

Trees, the works of God's own hand,
Tell the glory that is His—
Enrich the earth on which they stand,
But you are greater far than this.

A tree just grows in height and girth—
You grow in wisdom and in worth.

My biography appeared in *Who's Who in the Midwest*, seventh edition, and *Who's Who of American Women*, first and second editions.

I have also received the following honors: I was named "Missouri Nurse of the Year" in 1967 and received the All State Gold Medal Award. On the back of it was engraved "Vida E. Butterworth, R.N.—respected counselor, excellent organizer, server of the sick and heavy laden."

In 1971 I was honored by the Alumnae Association along with Miss Nelle Morgan for outstanding contributions to nursing education.

In January 1973 I received a certificate as a "Volunteer of the Year" from the Voluntary Action Center for work in the Northeastern Jackson County Mental Health Center where I had served since June 1971, helping to start a day activity center, organizing the library, being statistician for the center, and providing other specialized services.

I was honored by the Independence Branch of the American Association of University Women as "Woman of Achievement" for 1975 for community service at the Mental Health Center.

In 1976 I was selected as the winner of the "Outstanding Clubwoman" contest sponsored by the *Independence Examiner.*

The Alumnae Association of the Independence Sanitarium and Hospital School of Nursing presented me a beautiful pin for twenty-five years of service to the San School of Nursing. Later they gave me a plaque with this inscription: "The Alumnae Association of the Independence Sanitarium and Hospital School of Nursing hereby confers upon Vida E. Butterworth, R.N., this award of appreciation for forty-one years of devoted and meritorious service, acknowledging distinguished service to professional nursing, the hospital, the school of nursing, the Alumnae Association and the sponsoring church."

Since retirement I have kept busy with various volunteer services for various social organizations, but I do miss the challenge of student nurses and the feeling of satisfaction that comes from accomplishment commensurate with time and effort put forth.

ON RECORD

AFFILIATIONS

Back in my student days the only affiliation we had was in pediatrics at Children's Mercy Hospital in Kansas City, Missouri. At first it was four months and students were assigned to the baby ward, isolation, medical and surgical ward, orthopedics, boys' and girls' ward, and outpatient clinics. I found it a rather frightening experience because "the powers" were strict, nonyielding, and prone to "bawl out" students in public situations. In addition, most of us feared that we might be expelled for infringement of some rule that we didn't even know existed.

While at Mercy Hospital we attended classes taught by a pediatrician and had to write a pediatric case study. In more recent times the students have had excellent courses in pediatric nursing, child growth, and development (at least twenty hours, including many ward classes conducted by the students themselves). These classes have been taught by pediatric nurses and specialists in various pediatric areas. Most students enjoyed caring for the children, liked their teachers and supervisors, and gained much from their classwork and clinical experience. In later years this affiliation was for only three months.

Students lived in the dormitory while at Children's Mercy Hospital. Eventually there was a student council and each school had a representative attend council meetings to plan activities for the students on affiliation.

As soon as we obtained a full-time chaplain at the San (between 1948 and 1950) each group on affiliation from the San was visited by the chaplain and his wife who took all of the students out to dinner and a movie. This was always a red-letter day for the girls. (Students of other schools couldn't see why they were not provided this same courtesy.)

The next affiliations that were arranged for San students involved a choice between eight weeks of visiting nursing or three months of psychiatric nursing at St. Louis, Missouri. Those who chose visiting nursing seemed to enjoy it very much. Eventually this had to be discontinued because the Visiting Nurse Association excluded all students except those in collegiate programs. About this time the Missouri State Board of Nursing also made the three months experience in psychiatric nursing mandatory for all students in the state.

Most of the San students did well in psychiatric nursing and we could see when they came back that they were much better nurses because they could deal constructively with their patients' mental and emotional problems. Since they were permitted to have counseling at St. Louis State Hospital while on affiliation, many of them learned how to handle their own problems or anxieties in a more mature way.

At first we had some difficulty when the students who

had been on affiliation in St. Louis told the other students who hadn't been there all the "horror stories" concerning psychotic patients. We finally eliminated this through group counseling. The faculty, the chaplain, and the seniors who had been on affiliation met with the juniors who were about to go and discussed the experience. The faculty and chaplain encouraged a realistic discussion and suggested that the seniors talk about the positive values rather than the sensational experiences.

The next affiliation set up was for tuberculosis nursing. At first this was for eight weeks at Koch Hospital in St. Louis. This hospital was located at the edge of the city and students had to take a long bus ride to get "downtown" to a movie or to see friends. In the winter, San students were often the only ones there on affiliation and found the experience rather lonely. Those affiliating during the warmer months enjoyed the freedom of spacious surroundings, the Missouri River, and the rustic life. This affiliation was later changed to the Missouri State Tuberculosis Sanatorium at Mt. Vernon. Nearby Saints often took the students to church, invited them out to eat on Sunday, and provided some social activities that also included groups of patients.

The last few years of the San school most of the students had orientation with Public Health Nursing at the Jackson County Health Department. Here they obtained a smattering of the principles of public health nursing. After graduation many worked for the Visiting Nurse Association of Kansas City, the Jackson County Health Department, the Independence Health Department, the Kansas City or Independence Boards of Education as school nurses, or for private industry as industrial nurses. In fact, a number of them became supervisors or directors of public health nursing agencies.

The affiliation program at the San was one of the most extensive in the state of Missouri. Because of all these experiences San graduates had a wide range of skills. They had learned to get along with instructors, supervisors, and directors of other institutions and knew more than one way to do nursing procedures. The affiliation programs broadened and deepened their educational experiences and made them better able to cope with life as well as helping them to become successful nurses.

CHAPLAINS

When I came to the San there was no full-time chaplain. Usually the Stone Church pastor either conducted the 6:45 a.m. Chapel in the hospital dining room or appointed someone else to do it.

Later Patriarch Roy V. Hopkins (retired) served as part-time chaplain and was responsible for Chapel services; he also met many of the patients' needs for ministerial services.

Between 1948 and 1950 Donald V. Lents was appointed to serve as the first full-time chaplain at the hospital. He was under general church appointment and responsible to the First Presidency. Chaplain Lents had an office on the fifth floor of the new (1943) San. He was responsible for the nurses' chapel services. He also visited all patients in the morning prior to their surgery and administered to those desiring it. He was a member of the Hospital Board of Trustees, the School of Nursing Committee, and the faculty (he taught a religion class that was part of the curriculum). He helped to select the students who applied for entrance. This led to a standing joke. When he had Admission Committee meetings to go over applications and to select the students who would be entering the school, we looked closely at the grades and the health records, but we accused Chaplain Lents of looking at the photographs. If the girl was beautiful, he'd say, "She meets my qualifications. I vote for her." Seriously, he was helpful because he knew so many people throughout the country where he had been under appointment. He often knew the parents and sometimes even the prospective student.

Another of his duties was to counsel student nurses and hospital employees. As faculty sponsor for the Student Worship Committee he helped to plan Religious Emphasis Days to which college students of the area and RLDS young people wherever they might be in college were invited. This was held once or twice a year at various college campuses and sometimes at the San Recreation Building. The chaplain and his wife always chaperoned the student nurses when the meeting was out of town. Religious Emphasis Days gave the girls an opportunity to meet college students of their own age.

Another thing the chaplain did was to have an elective religion class in the early evening once a week. Not all girls coming to the San School of Nursing were of the RLDS religion, but some were converted while in the school.

Chaplain Lents was replaced by Almer Sheehy who

served 1951 through 1954. Almer was so vivacious, humorous, and outgoing that he too made a wonderful chaplain. His work with the students was supplemented by his wife Vivian and their three sons who attended many of the extracurricular activities.

Ray Ashenhurst was chaplain from 1954 to 1958. He was a quiet though forceful influence among the student nurses as he went about his duties.

Robert Farnham came in 1959 and remained until 1965. His contagious smile added much to faculty meetings and student religious activities. About this time student nurses were permitted to marry and remain in the school if they had the permission of their parents and the School of Nursing Committee, the faculty, and had premarriage counseling by the chaplain. He not only gave good advice but served as a beautiful example.

Soon the need for additional hospital chaplains arose, so Brother Farnham undertook to teach retired Independence priesthood members to function as assistants. In this way there would be chaplains available at all hours.

Leland Negaard acted as chaplain from 1965 to 1968. As was the case with all of the previous chaplains, he found his time taken up by School of Nursing and hospital duties.

Donald Harvey came in 1969 and served until the school closed in 1971. He did much to build up the chaplaincy staff and did a great deal of individual as well as group counseling in the newly organized alcohol unit of the hospital. During his chaplaincy the Hospital Chapel, financed by the San Nurses' Alumnae Association, was built. Services are held there each Sunday at

10:00 a.m. for patients who are able to walk there or come by means of crutches, wheelchairs, or perambulators.

The chapel is the San Alumnae's crowning achievement.

CLASSROOMS

Classrooms were located in many places—at the Sanitarium, at the Campus, at the Nurses' Residence, and finally in a separate Educational Building.

When I was a student we had no classrooms as such. An empty room or ward served the purpose, and in pleasant weather classes were often held out on the lawn or on the roof of the old hospital.

For a time the porch of first floor at the old 1215 West Van Horn Road Nurses Residence was used as a temporary classroom and nursing laboratory.

Between 1932 and 1935 a large classroom was set up in the basement. This contained about thirty chairs, one hospital bed unit, two bookcases, a procedure tray cupboard, and a piano. Chapel was held there after breakfast five mornings a week. I used to pray for a classroom without a piano so we'd have more room for nursing. After 1935 classrooms were set up in the basement of the new hospital. A nutrition laboratory was later established in Will Smith's workshop (where hospital equipment was repaired and new furniture was built).

After the first three floors of the new hospital were

completed, classrooms were moved to fourth floor of the new building.

Finally, after the collection of San Day Funds from 1949 until 1960 a one-story Educational Building was completed. This was "bliss on earth." We had instructors' offices in the basement of the hospital building and later in the Nurses Residence. Other facilities included a large nursing laboratory, a medicine room, a utility room, and a classroom where students were taught o.r. technique.

The new Educational Building housed a large library with study tables and chairs, a librarian's office, a conference room, a large classroom with armchair seating for sixty students, plus visual aids to help in teaching, a large science laboratory, and offices for an instructor, the educational director, and the school secretary. There was also an assembly room in the 1943 hospital used for a classroom.

Late in the history of the school a ward classroom was built on second floor of the hospital. It was a very good addition to the educational program and was used by the hospital personnel as well as the School of Nursing.

The School of Nursing was located at 1505 and 1509 West Truman Road when it was closed in 1971.

LIBRARY

When I entered the school of nursing the only library we had was located at the nurses' home. In the back parlor there was a big old bookcase with glass doors; in it were some really old books. Two of them—*Nursing*

Ethics and *Nursing Textbook*—were copyrighted in the 1890s.

What few texts we had we bought—*Nursing, History of Nursing, Anatomy and Physiology, Psychology, Materia Medica, The Mathematics of Drugs and Solutions.* These cost about $2.50 apiece. In most classes we had lectures by doctors, Miss Grapes, and Miss Copeland; we took notes and studied these for final tests.

When I became an instructor in August 1935, I found the same antiquated books at the nurses' home. No one had disturbed them. By now I knew the value of these books from the historical viewpoint and appropriated them to start our historical collection.

Having been at college with its separate library building which had a whole floor of books about nursing, I knew how valuable such reference material was. I knew it was important to get more than one person's viewpoint on any subject, and I longed for a modern library for the San school.

When Miss Copeland was going to the National Hospital Convention and asked me what I would like her to bring me I replied, "Please, bring me books for the school library." She brought two—*The Life of Florence Nightingale* and *The Conquest of Mexico.*

The next year when she went to the convention she again asked, "What shall I bring you?" I replied, "Please bring me some books about nursing," and she snapped, "I brought you two books last year. What more do you want?" I replied, "I want a School of Nursing Library."

I continued to solicit books. I received samples from

publishers and some volumes from the doctors; others I purchased myself. When I went to a nursing convention with its displays, the first thing I did was to visit all the book booths and carefully examine every new offering. If I had money—the school's or my own—for books, I made comparisons and tried to choose the ones that would best meet the students' needs.

In 1943 Miss Copeland and Miss Morgan asked Mrs. George Tousley, a hospital volunteer, to catalog our books and set up a functioning library. Mrs. Tousley accepted and immediately began to study library science. She became one of the best librarians in the area. After she had cataloged our meager supply she became interested in acquiring more and better books for the library.

After "San Day" was initiated, a definite amount of money per student was budgeted annually for the library. Besides that, each girl was charged a small fee which went to pay the expenses of the library. Before this no money was budgeted for this purpose. Mrs. Tousley paraphrased a noted actress who said, "I don't know any man with a thousand dollars, but I do know one thousand men with a dollar each." She capitalized on this idea and asked people to contribute at least one dollar a year to help finance the library; these people were called contributing patrons. The two little rooms that had been built by enclosing the west porch had all their bookshelves filled.

When the dining room was moved to the new building the light and spacious old dining room became the library. The old tables were refinished and used as reading tables. This remained the library until completion of the Education Building which contained a librarian's office, a huge area for stacks and reading tables, and a conference room with stacks for periodicals and the historical library. The librarian began receiving a small salary. At times students supervised the library in the evening for pay. In addition to Mrs. Tousley, those who have served as librarians or assistants through the years have been Doris Weddle, Myrtle Quitmyer, Jill Spencer, Sharon Powell, and Vinnie Hatch.

After Graceland students began coming to the San for nursing experience a librarian with a library science degree was appointed; Eric Campbell was the first to serve (1969 to 1971). The present librarian is Grace Ebeling. The facility is now known as "The Charles F. Grabske Memorial Library." Dr. Grabske devoted much time to the education of student nurses.

NURSES RESIDENCES

A word picture of the housing provided for the San students throughout the years will bring back many memories for those who attended the school of nursing.

Before 1926 nurses had lived on the third floor of the hospital because not all of the beds were needed for patients. In "my" day and until the 1940s the main residence was 1215 Van Horn Road (now Truman Road). We understood that at one time it had been an old folks home. It housed the hospital superintendent, Gertrude Copeland; assistant superintendent of nurses, Elizabeth Jane Paxton; the housemother, Mrs. Sarah

Thomas; and from twenty-four to thirty-four student nurses.

Most of us slept on the first- or second-floor sleeping porches. In the winter we kept woolen blankets, flannel gowns, caps, wool socks, and robes on the radiators to get them hot. At night we'd dress in all these "warmed" things and plunge quickly into bed. Many times in the winter when we were awakened by the six o'clock bell we'd have to shake the snow off our covers before getting up. Fortunately most of us were used to sleeping in unheated rooms at home. I have one thing to say for it: the common cold was far less prevalent among the student nurses then than in later years when students slept in heated quarters.

Other nurses' residences were used in the 1930s. At that time there were thirty to forty girls in the school.

In 1943 the students moved onto first floor of the old hospital building. It housed both the day and night residence directors, the director of nursing, the educational director, the operating room supervisor, and twenty-three students.

In 1944 the house at 1034 West Lexington became a residence for thirteen nurses and the educational director served as housemother. I believe they had a closer relationship, more cooperative study, more worship experiences, and more fun than any other group at the San.

We had many candy parties, hamburger fries, and potlucks in this residence because it was quite a way to walk back to the hospital to eat in the dining room at suppertime. I think everyone felt a warm, loving relationship in the group.

One night a student came in late. She waited in the hallway expecting a reprimand from me. When none came she sneaked in quietly and went to her room. Days went by and she wondered when she would be called on the carpet. She thought the "punishment of waiting" was the worst she had ever had. She did not realize until weeks later, when she told me about it, that I had never known she had come in late.

The residence at 1413 West Truman Road, across the street from the old hospital, also was used as a nurses' residence. Gertrude Copeland and her mother lived on first floor and the students lived on second. Mrs. Copeland acted as housemother until her death; then Miss Copeland (retired by that time) became housemother.

Still later a house back of the hospital was used by some of the seniors. For a year or two an instructor lived with them. Later, to conserve space, the students living there were especially chosen by the faculty and placed on their honor to live there without supervision. They handled this responsibility very well.

Sometimes a new class arrived before all of the students from the graduating class had completed their courses. This meant that there was not dormitory space for everyone. When this happened the students were allowed to "live out" and the hospital paid their rent until they completed their course.

Students have stayed in a number of places. The "dorm" was where a lot of them talked over their joys, sorrows, problems, inspirations, and plans for the future with other nurses. Those residences witnessed "a lot of living."

RECREATIONAL FACILITIES

I had been agitating since 1935 for a place that the students might call their own to use for shows, parties, sports, and religious activities—a place where they could cook and serve refreshments.

We usually had San School of Nursing parties in the dining room of the San or at the Stone Church. One night in the early 1930s the student nurses were permitted to use the "Playhouse" at Dr. G. L. Harrington's for a student activity. It was very adequate for many of the nurses' functions. After that every time we had a School of Nursing Committee meeting or one at which Gertrude Copeland met with the faculty or students I discussed how nice it would be to have a recreational building for the students. I talked with Nelle Morgan, members of the Hospital Board of Directors, and staff doctors (individually and collectively).

Finally in 1953 the Recreation Building (a steel auditorium with full stage) became a reality due to the efforts of the School of Nursing Committee and the Hospital Board of Trustees, especially Brother L. F. P. Curry, who made arrangements for the purchase of the building. It was erected south of the old hospital building at a cost of $35,000. On November 19 and 20 it was dedicated with a history of nursing pageant titled "Heritages and Horizons," produced for the community. The pageant was written by Myrtle Quitmyer. Student nurses and hospital personnel portrayed the historical characters in full costume. Lois Williams Daniels (hospital records librarian) directed the play. Mabel Faulkner and I designed and made most of the costumes. They were quite authentic because the History of Nursing class had researched pictures and descriptions to help. In fact, for this I had dressed dolls in authentic costumes and had kept them on display around the school and hospital.

We sewed for days, making the costumes and fitting them to the individuals who would wear them. Rehearsals were time-consuming but constructive. Everyone wanted the pageant to be a worthwhile and memorable occasion. And indeed it was. So the Recreation Building was off to a flying start.

I am sure that the Rec Building helped to preserve the sanity of both student nurses and instructors. It was a place where excess energy could be drained off in socially accepted ways—wrestling (mats provided), table tennis, basketball, volleyball, etc.

Later the Rec Building was destroyed by fire produced by neighborhood children who dropped lighted matches in a woodpile outside a window. This caught the curtains and the stage drapes on fire. The building was rebuilt as soon as possible.

Productions within this facility were colored by the creativity of the nurses. They became international with the arrival of students from Canada, England, Hawaii, and Vietnam. Some outstanding performances were held there and on the hospital lawn. I remember a spring festival with the theme, "Spring in Many Lands." At that time a dance instructor taught the girls the dances of various countries, including the highland fling, Mexican hat dance, and Dutch clog. Authentic costumes were made for each participating nurse and faculty member. Even the waitresses and salesmen in booths were in native dress. There were concession stands, gypsy fortune-tellers, a wishing well, an ice cream parlor, a hot dog stand, photograph booth, cake walk, and ducking pond.

At some of these festivals as much as $1,000 would be cleared in a single night because of the loyalty of the students and townspeople.

The Rec Building enabled us to hold many extracurricular activities, including the following:

1. Variety shows, written and put on by students with faculty help
2. Original plays and old-fashioned "Melodrammers"
3. Folk dances
4. Volleyball and basketball games
5. Carnivals
6. Parties
7. Religious Emphasis Day meetings

COSTS AND COST ANALYSIS

When I entered the School of Nursing I had to pay fifty dollars to cover expenses and furnish my own uniforms and duty hose. After three months probationary period I received an allowance of seven dollars a month. (I don't know what other students used their allowance for, but usually I spent mine for shoes and hose. We walked many miles up and down those hospital corridors for six to twelve hours a day.) I don't think I could have made it through training without that meager income.

As the years went by expenses at the School of Nursing increased. Students had to have more books and the cost of each went up. When I started teaching in 1935 most textbooks cost about $2.50 apiece. When the school closed in 1971 they cost between $12.50 and $17.50. The cost of food, suitable living quarters, and salaries also went up. Consequently the cost of a nursing education at the San rose.

In 1949, according to the auditor's report, the total cost of the School of Nursing was $39,667.20. That figures out to about $736.33 per student. Of this sum the student paid either in hours of work or cash. Actually at that time the student paid in fees, tuition, etc., $514.00, and the value of her services averaged $328.09, or a total for one year of $842.10. That would make the approximate cost for the full three years, $2,208.99. Thus each student would pay in service $984.27 and $1,542.03 in actual fees.

To show how things changed through the years I shall quote costs and figures from July 1, 1968, through June 30, 1969. There was an average enrollment of 106.75 students during that period. The total cost of the school was $403,889.94 for one year with $3,783.51 per student. During that year all of the students worked a total of 27,347 days in the hospital; these services were worth $35,023.34. Students paid $54,870.70 for tuition, fees, and supplies. The total income paid by students to the hospital in service and actual money was $89,894.04, or $842.10 per student. The deficit between the cost and what the student paid in money and service was $2,099.31. This deficit in 1968-69 was met by San Day funds of $25,853.38 and by World Church Conference appropriation for raising salaries of Nursing School faculty of $20,000. Later federal funds of $5,560 were received to help defray this expense.

As the cost of maintaining the hospital and the School of Nursing rose through the years so did the cost to the patient. The cost of teaching students also increased. The quality of service also went up because of new equipment such as the heart monitor and defibrillator and improved diagnostic tools.

In order to use this lifesaving equipment doctors and students had to have a more sophisticated education. These costs increased commensurate with the rise in the cost of living. For instance, when I came in training hospital costs to the patient were as follows:

Wards—$2.00 per day
Semiprivates—$3.00 per day
Ordinary private rooms—$4.00 per day
Special private rooms—$5.00 per day.

In 1941:

Wards—$4.00 per day
Two-bed rooms—$5.00 per day
Private rooms—$6.00 per day
Private rooms with two windows—$6.50 per day
Private rooms with bath—$7.50 per day

Recently the *Independence Examiner* carried an announcement that the Independence Sanitarium and Hospital was dropping the costs of hospital care $8.00 per day. That is two-thirds of what a ward bed cost for an entire week back in 1926.

CURRICULUM AND EXTRACURRICULAR PROGRAMS

As educational director I was responsible for the formulation of the curriculum for the School of Nursing and also the extracurricular program. Before 1931 nurses had some nursing classes, ethics, hospital housekeeping, bacteriology, and chemistry taught by an RN, but most of the nursing procedures were taught by older student nurses to younger ones.

Many courses such as anatomy, physiology, materia medica, medicine, surgery, eye-ear-nose-and-throat, gynecology, emergency, dermatology, obstetrics, psychiatry, and neurology were taught by the physicians who practiced in the hospital. Most of our classes were taught in the dining room. We sat about the tables and chewed up toothpicks while the doctors lectured, interrupting them occasionally with questions. These dining room lecturers were Dr. John R. Green, Dr. C. H. Allen, Dr. Calvin Atkins, Dr. W. Hobbs, Dr. Stanley L. Green, Dr. Tom Twyman, Dr. Stuart Gillmore, Dr. Charles Krimminger, and Dr. Charles Keown. Psychiatry, neurology, and dermatology were taught at one of the city hospitals (usually at Research Nurses' Home) by Dr. G. L. Harrington, Dr. Landis B. Elliott, and Dr. Charles Dennie.

By 1936 San seniors were attending St. Luke's and Trinity Lutheran Hospitals also, where they had lectures in sociology, survey of the nursing field, and professional adjustments. These were twice a week for eight or nine months. At the end of each section tests were given and graded by an instructor who sponsored and supervised students at the classes. The girls enjoyed making the trip to Kansas City and meeting seniors from other schools. Often they were associated with these students later while on affiliation in psychiatric, pediatric, tuberculosis, and visiting nursing.

Students had approximately 500 hours of classwork. They attended September through May, with vacations in the summer.

In the late 1950s the curriculum was revised so that the classwork and the clinical experience were concurrent. Some classes that were not clinically oriented, however, ran all through a semester or year. There were also many hours of patient-oriented ward teaching in which the dietitian, doctors, graduates, and students cooperated so that patient needs could be met.

A listing of actual subject matter might better indicate the nursing program at this stage. Classes were divided into fourths, each with its own clinical rotation and matching classes being taught to these small groups only. There was also a core of studies (not clinical) that all four quarters of the class attended at the same time. Here is the 1960 curriculum:

First year

Anatomy, physiology, biochemistry, and pathology	124 hours
Chemistry, inorganic and organic	80 hours
Microbiology	64 hours
Foundations of nursing	214 hours
Community field trips and social aspects	48 hours

Psychology	70 hours
Sociology	32 hours
Mathematics of drugs and solutions	20 hours
First Aid	28 hours
Pharmacology I	33 hours
Pharmacology II	16 hours
Pharmacology III	6 hours
Nutrition, foods, and cookery	50 hours
Clinical nutrition (diet therapy)	72 hours
Obstetric nursing	60 hours
Basic medical nursing	90 hours
Surgical nursing	95 hours
Operating room nursing	95 hours
Second year	
History of nursing	18 hours
Comparative religions	24 hours
Professional adjustments	41 hours
Advanced medical-surgical nursing (including ward teaching and management)	95 hours
Tuberculosis nursing	60 hours
Third year	
Pediatric nursing	82 hours
Psychiatric nursing	120 hours
Senior lectures	66 hours
Communication	6 hours

By 1971 the hours had in some cases been added to and in other cases cut down in individual subjects, but they were reduced to 1,090 hours of class in the total program and a great many of these were clinical ward classes, held not just for the good of the student nurses but for the total benefit of all nursing personnel on the ward; they were particularly geared to helping the nursing staff aid the individual patients studied.

The following brief summary shows better what was involved in teaching at the San from the inception of the school:

1912 - 1 graduate
1920 - 8 graduates, 21 classes
1928 - 9 graduates, 24 classes, 730 hours
1939 - 12 graduates, 27 classes, 1,090 hours
1948 - 1951 - 17 graduates, 31 classes, 779 hours
1957 - 1959 - 32 graduates, 32 classes, 1,745 hours
1963 - 1965 - 34 graduates, 26 classes, 1,931 hours
1967 - 1968 - 34 graduates, 16 classes, 1,704 hours
1971 - 27 graduates, 27 classes, 1,457 hours

As educational director I was chairman of the faculty. Together we made out the curriculum and assigned the subjects to the various instructors. We had (when the school was the largest) sixteen full-time and six part-time instructors.

Much of my work was done in conjunction with the faculty or committees. The accrediting Self-Evaluation Study had to be done by schools wanting national accreditation. This required discussions with the school faculty and representatives of the affiliative agencies where students studied and received experiences in the nursing of children, psychiatric patients and people with chronic lung diseases, visiting, and public health nursing.

Sometimes faculty meetings brought out some rather heated discussions that lasted until we could come to a decision satisfactory to all.

The first school catalog was published about 1920; it contained little information and no pictures. The next one was a combined hospital yearbook and catalog published in 1928. I remember it had a photograph of my class (1929) and other pictures as well as a summary of the school curriculum.

The next catalog was published after I started teaching. It was not dated so that we could use it for a number of years. Some time in the 1940s, however, we began publishing a new catalog every two or three years so it would be up-to-date. It described the current curriculum, expenses, equipment needed, school rules and regulations, etc. Whenever a new one was to be printed, the faculty spent hours going over the current catalog bringing it up-to-date.

I had overall charge of the student organization, student council, and extracurricular activities; however, each committee of the organization and each branch of student activity also had a faculty sponsor. Faculty members were kept busy ten to fourteen hours a day. Most of them enjoyed their work and supervising recreation, so there were few problems.

When I first came back to the San to teach after getting my M.S. degree I realized more than before how much the students needed a place for organized recreation. Eventually an oven was built on the east lawn of the nurses residence. Here the girls had weiner roasts, hamburger fries, breakfasts cooked in the open, picnics, and ice cream socials. At least three attempts were made to provide tennis courts. When I was a student there was a makeshift court at the west end of the old hospital. It was not used often because the nurses were on their feet so much that swift footwork was not appealing as a form of recreation.

Later a court was built southwest of the old San in what used to be the "garden plot." Again there was not much time for tennis except before 6:00 a.m. and after 7:00 p.m. Interest lagged and the court eventually grew up in weeds.

Still later one was built west of the Recreation Building. It was surrounded by a high fence to keep the balls in and the neighborhood children out. It, too, eventually fell into disuse and became a part of the hospital parking lot.

Student nurses always needed money for their various projects, and they earned it in many ways. One was "Tagday" when students in uniform stood on prominent street corners in Independence and solicited for a "free bed" at the hospital.

Sanilog, the school yearbook, was first published in 1930 by the "San Centennial" class. Not until 1946 did it become a regular production. Members of each *Sanilog* staff felt their particular book was *the* outstanding one. Each book was dedicated to a particular person or group that the *Sanilog* staff felt deserved special honor.

The students also published a monthly newspaper for many years. It sort of went by starts and stops according to the whims of the editorial staff and writers. At first it was named *The ISH*. Later it became *The Portico* (entrance to the 1943 hospital). By reading these school publications one could determine the morale of the student body at any particular time.

Other projects for which the students raised money through the years included the following:

1. Purchasing a grand piano for the Student Nurses' Lounge.
2. Paying a $2,000 pledge on the hospital drive. (Students did this by working one day for the hospital and contributing their salaries to the building fund.)
3. Refurnishing the student lounge with furniture they themselves chose at a cost of $1,000.
4. Paving a tennis court and purchasing needed sports equipment.
5. Building a swimming pool in front of the Nurses' Residence (surrounded with a redwood fence).

After the School of Nursing was closed the pool was taken over by the hospital and used to give swimming lessons to the children in the Hospital Day Care Center, for hospital personnel swimming parties, and on the day of the "all-hospital picnic" when employees were treated to a free picnic lunch and supper on the grounds of the old San.

It was a sorry day when the swimming pool, a big walnut tree, and a beautiful pin oak were removed so the area could be turned into an asphalt-covered parking lot for physicians. Some of us "old-timers" stood on the front porch and wept as we saw our work and God's handiwork being destroyed.

Many students went back to their own or different cities. On the basis of their curricular and extracurricular activities while in the School of Nursing they functioned well in various community, church, school, and recreational programs.

DISCIPLINE THROUGH THE YEARS

In 1921 (the first record I can find) student rules and regulations were made by the School of Nursing Committee.

When I was working on third floor, someone left a baby on the table in the nursery without supervision. (The rule was that babies must be kept in their cribs except when a nurse was working directly with them.) When discovered the baby had a reddened area which everyone feared might be burned enough to raise a blister. All student nurses on the maternity floor were suspected. To be sure that the real culprit received punishment each nurse had her cap taken away. This was to last until an investigation was made and the real culprit could be determined and punished. I removed my cap and went back to work. Some of the other students wanted to refuse to accept the punishment, but I said, "I'll not do that. I'll take the punishment even though I know I was not responsible."

We were taken one at a time to the Battery Block Building uptown and questioned by G. L. Harrington. If he ever found the guilty person the rest of us never knew it. The next day we were told we might wear our caps again. I was relieved to know that I was not to be "kicked out" of training.

When students made low grades they were forced to spend certain hours each evening in supervised study. This, however, proved to be harder on the instructor supervising than to the students, so it was not long enforced.

Campusing was another favorite punishment for infringement of rules. Usually that meant students couldn't leave the hospital and Nurses Home for one or two weeks.

Other discipline included adding days to the nursing course for such things as chewing gum on duty, being late to work, and bobbing hair (that was in 1926).

In the middle forties a student-faculty association was formed to help maintain high morale. A student council with representatives from all three classes, committee chairmen for all student activities, and two faculty members met biweekly.

Duties of the student-faculty organization were as follows:

1. To foster cooperation and good fellowship among students.
2. To facilitate friendly relations between faculty and students.
3. To plan extracurricular activities both within the school and among schools of nursing in the Kansas City area.
4. To foster the establishment and maintenance of scholastic and social standards in the School of Nursing.

In 1959 this became known as the Student Body Organization. Students assumed more responsibility for themselves and each other on a merit system. A student and the residence director did weekly inspection of rooms together. Punishments were set up by the students for not cleaning the recreation area after using it and for not keeping rooms cleaned. Discipline was established by the merit board consisting of several students and one faculty member. Students were often harder on each other than the faculty would have been. There were many outstanding student body presidents during the years I was educational director. In fact, in one way or another each was outstanding. All became efficient in planning and carrying out various student activities. We were very proud of their successes.

FACULTY

The Sanitarium has been very fortunate in having good instructors for the School of Nursing.

The first was Jennie Weed Hahn. Mary Wise Moats also did some teaching. San graduates who have served as instructors are as follows: May Richards Cook Ham (1917), Elsie Barnett Wombles (1914), Laura Mann Bateman (1916), Catherine Stephens Alexander (1923), Faye Franklin (1921), Eva Franklin (1924), Ina Hattey Smith (1924), Myrtle Grapes Quitmyer (1924), Jennie Cochran Linkhart (1930), Iola Rogers Campbell (1927), Shirley Butler (1930), Nelle Morgan (1930), Mabel Andrew McKevitt (1931), Mabel Faulkner (1932), Stella Eskridge Earnshaw (1934), Eula Baughman Allen (1940), Nina Propst Hartley (1941), Annella Lou Butler

(1943), Marjorie Stobaugh Trinkle (1953), Marilyn Wismer Kettlewell (1954), Lois Rounds Spencer (1956), Evelyn Directo Jordan (1957), Gayla Meadows Siy (1960), Margaret Walker Rowe (1948), Marna Etter Burgess (1961), Lucy Ann Laur Fleischman (1961), Elaine Lenox Thompson (1947), Peggy Dellar Eslinger (1954), Lucy Marie Nelson Land (1937), Ruth Jones Haukenberry (1943), Olena Elaine Epperson (1937), Ella Winholtz (1937), Beryle Jean Closson Immer (1966), Betty Hutchins Trimble (1946), Joyce Richardson Shireman (1952), Carlotta Ballantyne Sinclair (1946), Nancy Arvilla Pement Weldon (1952), Marja Parker Waldon (1961), Nancy McWilliams Stickel (1962), Lucille Gress (1954), Nancy Harter Krahl (1967), Nancy Locke Farley (1945), Jean Bastow Taylor (1970), Dorcas Hentz Wilkinson (1964), Mary Jo Kittinger (1968), Kathleen Armstrong Bennett (1966), Jean Gerber Livingston (1958), Iola Tordoff (1947), Lottie Coleman Papenfus (1948), Florence Nowack Welch (1949), Betty Buckley Russell (1943), Helen Hinde Wade (1947), Barbara Gibson (1952), and Mary Ann Storm Good (1934).

At least sixty-five instructors were not San graduates; some chaplains, nutritionists, dietitians, etc., were not even nurses. These faculty members also contributed much to the education of the students.

San grads who taught elsewhere than the San are as follows: Edith Wingett (1934), Research Hospital in Kansas City; Merle North (1955), psychiatric nursing at a hospital in California; Linda Tripp Tedrow (1955), OB-parent classes at a hospital in Kansas; Diana Worthington (1956), pediatric diabetes at a hospital in

Wichita; Ila June Coon Brunner (1957), University of Nebraska at Omaha; Lavern Rogers (1957), hospital in Escatawpa, Mississippi; Barbara Thoman Curtis (1960), Washington State; Faye Ballantyne Busch (1961), psychiatric nursing at Western Missouri Mental Health Center; Beverly Smith Bechtel (1961), Trinity Lutheran in Kansas City; Lucille Gress (1954), Kansas University School of Nursing; Kathryn Madsen Houser (1934), hospital in Illinois; Rose Marie Hilker Oakes (1952), director of school of nursing at St. Luke's Hospital in Kansas City; Verna Watters Moreland (1948), director of nurses in a Missouri hospital; Iola Tordoff (1947), Kansas University Medical Center; Phyllis Norcross Lansberg (1961), director of nurses at the hospital in Lexington, Missouri.

After Pearl Harbor so many doctors went to the service that those remaining had no time to teach student nurses, so the number of nurse instructors increased at the San. At the same time the number of students increased because of the need for nurses and because the U.S. Cadet Nurse Corps insured a girl a nursing education without cost to her. Most instructors worked twelve to eighteen hours a day.

Miss Morgan, Miss Copeland, hospital administrators, and board members were always proud of the San graduates because wherever they went they were successful, adjustable, kind-hearted nurses wanting to do their best. San hospital administrators or directors of nurses often have met someone at a meeting or convention who has remarked on how San graduates have been hired when available and how acceptable their work has been. It certainly wasn't the location that made good nurses; it was the caliber of the student and the good teaching of the instructors. Experiences other than those in the classroom and ward helped to develop talents and abilities which enhanced the personality of the student nurse. Chapel Religious Emphasis Days, big and little sister programs, variety shows, plays, parties, and student organizations on the local, district, state, and national levels all helped. The San faculty also could always be counted on to spend the necessary hours to help round out the students' three years of experience.

As educational director I appreciated the devotion, creativity, long hours in the wards supervising students, the genuine interest in each individual student, and the arguments we had in faculty meetings trying to plan the most meaningful curriculum for all students. Always there was also concern about meeting each student's individual needs as much as possible.

SCHOOL OF NURSING COMMITTEE

The first committee of the Independence Sanitarium and Hospital Training School was appointed in 1921. This was made up of G. Leonard Harrington, M.D., Laura E. Mann, R.N., and Elizabeth J. Paxton, R.N. They dealt with such problems as these:

1. Taking away one student's three hours time off duty from September, 1920, to March 10, 1921, a total loss to the student of 573 off-duty hours.

2. Accepting three girls as probationers with one being accepted from a nurse attendant course with full credit.

3. Writing for educational records of three prospective students and character recommendations of another.

On September 7, 1921, the committee voted to teach the students according to standard curriculum for nurses. That was the year the Missouri State Board of Nursing became an entity and began to regulate the practice of nursing all over the state. The San school was state-accredited the first year accreditation went into effect. At that time students had a total of 236 hours of classwork in their three years of training and spent 52 hours a week in the hospital wards caring for patients.

Back on December 5, 1922, according to the School of Nursing Committee's minutes, Dr. Harrington and Miss Paxton met in the training school office and accepted a student just completing her three months probationary period. It was said that her work was not up to standard but that it had improved in the past month. This particular student seemed to have a paranoid-type reaction toward everything in general. They felt that if she could have sympathetic aid it would help her to do better work.

This girl did complete her nursing course and was a successful private duty nurse for many years.

The following note appeared in the school committee's minute book (looking as though it had been posted on a bulletin board):

Notice to Doctors, Nurses, and Our Friends

Miss Paxton and I are willing to donate $25.00 each toward a

reference library for the Training School.

How much will you give?

Laura E. Mann
Principal of the Training School

Another notice suggested that no long vacations could be had at Christmas and New Year's because it would be too hard to make up the classwork missed. Therefore, each girl would have the holidays off plus the Monday following but must attend classes on every other weekday after the holiday. Still another notice advised students that they must be responsible for any classes they might miss; the instructor could not be held accountable for the making up of classwork. The same was true if the student came in late after the semester started. Such students had to study harder and prepare for makeup examinations.

Apparently the committee, as such, died out at that time. Under Nelle Morgan's regime as director of the School of Nursing, another committee was organized on April 27, 1944, with the approval of the Board of Trustees of the hospital. The following are representative of subjects discussed at the first committee meeting:

1. a. Expansion of this committee.
   b. Budget for School of Nursing
   c. Recreation facilities
   d. Morning chapel
   e. Housing

2. It was agreed that the school should admit twenty to twenty-five students in September.

3. The consensus of opinion was that Vida Butterworth, educational director of the school, should be on the committee. President Smith was asked to write her a letter asking her to serve.

At the next meeting, May 25, 1944, these matters were discussed:

1. Prospective student applications were reviewed and nineteen students were accepted.

2. Military drill for students was recommended by the NLNE [for all students in the U.S. Cadet Nurse Corps]. Bishop DeLapp was appointed to make such arrangements with the local unit of the Missouri Infantry to start June 22, 1944.

4. The question of admitting Negro students was referred to Bishop DeLapp for answering.

5. The constitution and bylaws of the Student-Faculty Association were read and approved with a few minor changes.

At that time the School of Nursing had five committees: executive, recruitment, finance, residence, and nursing service. The constitution and bylaws were three pages in length.

This committee, with changes in personnel as needed, continued to function until the school was closed in 1971.

SCHOOL TRAGEDIES

Most institutions have had times of tragedy. The San School of Nursing was no exception. Probably the most tragic have been times when student nurses have died. The first to die at the San was Helen Logsdon, a victim of cerebrospinal meningitis in the early 1920s.

The next was Ardyce Eckart, who was to have been graduated with the class of 1930. She was out on a double date with another student when an accident occurred. Ardyce was brought to the San where it was discovered that a fractured rib had penetrated her liver. Within a few days Ardyce was dead.

At the graduation services during the Centennial Conference an empty chair was placed on the platform where the graduates were sitting. It was draped with a nurse's cape as if Ardyce were an invisible member of the class.

Connie Downs was a second-year student at the San when she went out one night on a date with her boyfriend. As they were coming home from Liberty (a little late) the boyfriend was speeding and missed the corner coming off the Missouri River Bridge on 291. The car rolled over, and Connie's neck was broken. She died instantaneously.

All of the students attended Connie's funeral and burial in uniform. At the cemetery her class formed a pathway from the hearse to the grave through which the casket was carried by the pallbearers.

The whole school was thrown into a state of depression by this tragedy for a while. The girls recovered before too long and resumed their normal life-style.

Student nurses grow up rapidly because they are confronted with life and death circumstances almost every day of their school and nursing experiences. We faculty members used to say that the girls entering the school in September seemed so young and immature. After Christmas, when they returned from their vacations, they were hardly recognizable as the same young women who had entered four months previously; the amount of maturity they had attained was almost unbelievable. Their interests were no longer the same. Of course, they loved their parents and wanted to see them, but after a few days at home they became restless and were anxious to get back to where the action was.

A fourth student who died while attending the school was Beverly Gates. A senior, she had her own Volkswagen. One of her best friends was being married in Mt. Pleasant, Iowa, and had asked Beverly to be a bridesmaid. To get there she had to drive over graveled roads. Her car skidded and overturned, killing her instantly. This, too, seemed an almost insurmountable tragedy and generated considerable depression among the students. But again they overcame their grief and took a monumental step toward mental and emotional health which made them much more understanding of how to handle such problems in bereaved persons with whom they would be associated.

While students encountered many tragedies—sudden illnesses, accidents, emergency operations, and death—they also had many joyous experiences. These ranged from the birth of a much-longed-for baby, recovery of a critically ill patient, and treats furnished by thankful patients and relatives.

There were usually high-level spiritual experiences occurring in chapel, the chaplain's services, and Religious Emphasis Days. These inspired them to give their best service in times of crises such as the Ruskin Heights tornado, the 1951 Missouri River flood, and the deep snow which prevented R.N.s from getting to work (students ran the hospital on an emergency basis). Such crises gave the students opportunity to practice their religion in a very practical way.

PLUSSES IN THE SAN NURSING PROGRAM

Highly emotional experiences of a positive nature were the feelings of success, satisfaction, and fulfillment that came with the nursing program. There was the publishing of *The Portico*, *The Sanilog*, and the holding of a May festival, a variety show, a carnival, a French café party, folk dances, and preparing floats for the annual Halloween parades.

There were, of course, both positive and negative emotions arising from tests, oral reports, group counseling sessions, educational and recreational movies, written reports, case studies, debates, term papers, and affiliation experiences away from the "home school."

Plusses of the San Nursing Program included the following:

1. Rotary scholarships for seven students
2. Etzenhouser student loan
3. Independence Jaycettes scholarship
4. Spellman Scholarship Fund
5. Annual San School of Nursing Day
6. Hurlbut Small Loan Fund (a student could borrow small amounts to be paid back when money was available)
7. Copeland Loan Fund (available to faculty members for college expenses)
8. Faculty grants with leave of absence to attend school. (These did not have to be repaid unless the receiver did not come back to the San and work for five years.)

9. Foreign professional students attending the San for additional education and supervised experience:
   a. Hoang Van Phi from Vietnam—three-year basic program
   b. Congtangton Na Minh Khuong—Vietnam—six weeks in medical-surgical nursing
   c. Hoand ding Bao—Vietnam—nursing administration for six weeks
   d. Salimo Ams—Basar, Iraq—six weeks nursing service
   e. Virginia Khamis—Ammon, Jordan—three months in nursing administration
10. Disaster planning—city-wide mock disaster practice
11. Prenatal classes for parents taught by Mabel Faulkner
12. Printed manuals for ward and student, such as
    a. Orthopedic manual
    b. House Order Book (kept updated)
    c. Experience record for students
    d. Diabetic manual
    e. Procedure manual
    f. Procedure checklist for students
    g. Patient care checklist for students
13. Student organizations with faculty sponsors
14. School of Nursing Chorus (local school and district nurses' association)
15. "Miss Student Nurse" Contest and annual speech contest
16. State Fair recruitment of students
17. Marriage and home-building courses for students and their boyfriends

18. Religious Emphasis Days
19. Annual hospital picnic
20. Alumnae Hawaiian luau
21. Annual alumnae bazaar and chili supper
22. Career teas
23. Hospital auxiliary
24. "Heritages and Horizons" (pageant on History of Nursing given at opening of Recreation Building)
25. New wing on second floor of hospital
26. Piped-in oxygen
27. *San Piper* (hospital newsletter)
28. Accredited School of Nursing, state board, national league for nursing
29. Community disaster drill
30. Participation in Center Stake volleyball game
31. Swimming pool
32. Student nurse representative on Zion's League Board
33. Rapid reading course provided at school expense
34. Monthly convocations
35. Leadership classes taught by representative seniors
36. School of Nursing Committee
37. Cataloged library
38. Celebration of twenty-fifth, thirty-fifth, fiftieth, and sixtieth anniversaries with community
39. Grade-point study made of Graceland students against non-Graceland students
40. Alumnae surveys made regularly every few years to show what graduates were doing (testing the products of the school)
41. Classes for diabetic patients

42. Classes for patients with respiratory difficulties

These plusses were the result of cooperation between faculty, school of nursing committee, hospital board of directors, hospital administration, and school administration.

OFF THE RECORD

In nursing and in hospital life we learn to face reality most of the time. There is laughter and happiness when a healthy baby is born; there are tears (either unshed or shed out of sight in a utility room) when someone dies. But taking the bitter with the sweet we know it averages out.

Soon all the nurses who acquired their knowledges and skills of nursing under "the old regime" will be gone and the new generation may think it was always as it is now. The fun we had can never be duplicated, because the era which allowed it has passed. The years have brought changes in so many things that we could never again have those types of experiences.

- - - - - - - -

Since so many amusing things happened to student nurses on and off duty, only a cross section can be recounted here. I recall one probie in the class of '32 who was asked to clean the thermometer tray. Since she wanted them to be especially sterile she boiled the thermometers. Since there is considerable difference between 110° and 212° F., the poor girl had to buy a whole new setup of thermometers.

When I was a probie, Dr. Charles H. Allen asked someone to describe the "acetabulum" (a part of the hip socket) in anatomy class. No one put up her hand to answer the question, so he asked each student in turn. His voice sounded threatening! I sat at the end of the row, and by the time he got to me I had figured out that what he was asking was what we had called the "a-seat-a-bellum." I answered correctly, and he gave me an all-out smile which amply repaid me for my hours of study (and for my astuteness in selecting an end seat).

Dr. Allen taught anatomy and physiology classes to freshman students for many years. He was an excellent instructor. I learned far more there than I did in one whole summer at Columbia University Medical Center. Most of the students were afraid of him. Underneath his rough exterior, however, he had a keen sense of humor and a real love for people. There was a special place in his heart for student nurses. (He had four daughters of his own, but none of them became doctors or nurses.)

Dr. Elmer Twyman was a prominent surgeon at the San as well as in Kansas City. Unfortunately he was often sarcastic with student nurses who assisted him during surgery. He always used one knife to cut the skin, but because the skin was considered contaminated (even though it had been painted with germicides) he always used another knife on the inner tissues. On one particular day the scrub nurse (who handed the instruments to the surgeon) had only one knife on the overpatient table. While he was waiting for a second, he asked the nurse, "Don't you know that a knife is as essential to the hand of a surgeon as a powder puff is to the hand of a flapper?" In the 1920s when "flappers" were all the rage, this said it all!

- - - - - - - -

We had some interesting lessons when we first started formal classes in the fall of 1926. I particularly remember my course in psychology taught by F. M. McDowell, Ph.D. He had a wonderful sense of humor and was delighted to learn of a very humorous happening at the San.

A certain young minister had surgery at the San. Because of his age, no one suspected him of having false teeth. The rule was that all false teeth had to be removed before the patient went to surgery, and that false teeth were to be kept in a special covered cup in the patient's bedside table.

This man went to surgery wearing his dentures, but the nurse returned them to his hospital room wrapped in a towel. Without reporting this to anyone, she left them on the bedside table. The nurse who came to clean his room while he was in surgery put the towel containing the dentures in with the soiled linen. Then the woman in charge of the linen room sent everything to the laundry uptown.

When an employee at the laundry found the dentures among the linen he immediately delivered them back to the linen room at the hospital. Here it was determined that they must belong to a woman who had died that day at the hospital. The relatives of the deceased had already taken her dentures to the undertaker, so the extra set was placed under her pillow in the casket.

In the meantime the minister returned to his room and inquired about his teeth. They were not to be found.

The anesthetist, who was also a dentist, made him a new set without charge.

All nurses were warned that this story must absolutely remain a secret, but somehow F. M. McDowell and John Sheehy heard about it.

Brother McDowell decided to find out how many really did know the story so he made an association test to demonstrate its use in the freshman psychology course. Six freshmen students took the test ostensibly to learn which ones had viewed a picture of a burning building showing firefighters, onlookers, and people who had apparently escaped from the burning building. Then he brought each of the six students before the class one at a time to say the first thing that came into their minds when test words were given. The three who had viewed the picture were easily picked out by their responses to the test words. Also, it was learned that all six taking the association test were in on the story of the missing false teeth. Every one responded to the key word in the test "false teeth" with the name of the person involved.

All of this goes to prove that rules are made for good reasons. *Never wrap dentures in a towel; place them in the cup especially made for them!*

- - - - - - - - -

Once the Independence police called Miss Copeland and said that neighbors had reported a dead body in the basement of the unfinished hospital. Miss Copeland tumbled immediately to the situation and invited the police out to view the "body."

She escorted them from her office on first floor of the old hospital down the stairs, through the basement of the old hospital, and into the "sheeted-off" nursing laboratory. There "in state" was Susie Chase, the nursing manikin. The police had a good laugh over that emergency call.

- - - - - - - -

This was a far cry from my probie days when I and other students of my vintage had to "lay out" a corpse just by following the directions in our hand-copied House Order Book, often without the aid of an older student nurse or R.N. Frequently this "laying out" was done in fear and trembling.

In later years each class of junior students had a four-hour seminar on death and dying taught by the chaplain, a nurse, a doctor, and a mortician. This seemed to help the students to accept the deaths of their patients with less emotional trauma. At the same time they were much better equipped to meet the needs of the bereaved.

- - - - - - - -

"Spinnie," one of the probies in my class, had a traumatic experience on night duty thought up by another fun-loving but irresponsible student. At 7:00 p.m. report the night nurses were informed that Mrs. M------- in 210 had died and her body was awaiting the undertaker. When the other student nurse on the ward went to supper, leaving "Spinnie" alone on the floor, another student went in 210, turned on the patient call signal, and hid under the bed.

When Spinnie saw the light on in the dead person's room she approached very cautiously and turned on the overhead light as she entered the room. The corpse was perfectly still under the white sheet, but Spinnie asked, "Did you want something?" The student nurse under the bed replied, "Nothing!" Spinnie was almost ready to jump out of her skin when the student came out from under the bed laughing. Spinnie said, "You almost made my heart stop beating. You'd better not try that again or I will report you to Miss Copeland." I never heard of it happening after that.

There was a lot of improvising done in the earlier days. I remember that in one classroom we bragged of having "running water." The students carried a bucket up to the faucet at the head of the tunnel, filled it, and ran all the way back to the classroom. Thus we could have running hot water for baths and enemas and cold water for drinking.

- - - - - - - -

Often the anatomy-physiology tests I gave students were twenty-some pages long. Many girls became overtense as they prepared to "dig in," so after they were all in the room I would have them stand in their places, take deep breaths, and *yell* at the top of their voices. This helped relieve tension and clear their brains for action, and I am sure many made higher grades than they would otherwise have made.

In 1942 Dr. Charles E. Grabske and I tried an experiment in the history of nursing class. Usually I was disappointed in the results of tests. I personally liked history of nursing so much that I couldn't comprehend how the students could help being fascinated by it and therefore remember it.

Benzedrine had just come on the market. It was supposed to improve one's memory. Dr. Grabske wrote me a prescription for one tablet for each student. I gave the tablets to the students one hour before time to take a repeat test. They hadn't done at all well on the first one. In fact I think there were several failures. The experiment came out as we had expected it to. Every student raised her grade point on the test at least one to two points, and some even more.

- - - - - - - -

There were different types of problems to face when I served as housemother at 1034 West Lexington. One day the sewer backed up into the basement. We were thirteen women alone, but we shoveled all the back flow into a garbage can and carried it out to the garden area, dug a deep hole, and buried it. Eleda Agur Smith (1947), who was the smallest, was put in the hole digging to make it deeper. We hosed down the basement and made the burial after dark.

Another time the furnace was giving us trouble. The bottom was full of large clinkers which we could not get out to keep the fire hot enough to warm the house, so we let the fire go out. When the furnace was cold we put tiny Eleda through the furnace door and had her hand out the large clinkers one by one. After getting her out and cleaned up we started the fire and soon had the house warm again. We were very self-sufficient.

- - - - - - - -

Another incident happened on Halloween. We were wanting to get rid of our nursing doll, "Mrs. Chase," who was equipped so nurses could practice baths, enemas, etc., on her. On this dark Halloween night a procession of student nurses and instructors carrying the manikin crossed Van Horn Road. They dug a hole behind the building that used to be where Resthaven is now and buried poor old "Susie." We always wondered if she showed up when the workmen were excavating for Resthaven.